Health and Social Services in Primary Care — an Effective Combination?

Edited by

Geoff Meads MA (Oxon) Msc
Professor of Health Services Development, Health Management Group, City University

With Foreword by

June Huntington
Independent Consultant and Visiting Fellow, King's Fund College

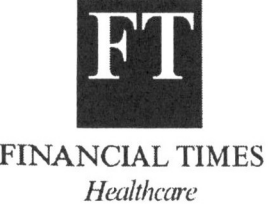

FINANCIAL TIMES
Healthcare

FT HEALTHCARE
a Division of Pearson Professional Ltd
Maple House, 149 Tottenham Court Road,
London W1P 9LL, UK
Telephone: +44 (0)171 896 2424
Fax: +44 (0)171 896 2449
http://www.fthealthcare.com

First published 1997

A catalogue record for this book is available from the British Library

ISBN 0-443-05911-X

© Pearson Professional Ltd 1997

All rights reserved. No part of this publication may be reproduced, stored in a retrieval system, or transmitted in any form or by any means, electronic, mechanical, photocopying, recording or otherwise without either the prior written permission of the publishers or a licence permitting restricted copying issued by the Copyright Licensing Agency Ltd, 90 Tottenham Court Road, London W1P 9HE.

Publisher: Mark Lane
Project Manager: Brenda Wren
Copy edited by: Patricia MacColl, Cupar
Indexed by: June Morrison, Helensburgh

Typeset by Saxon Graphics Ltd, Derby

Printed by Bell and Bain Ltd, Glasgow

Contents

Contributors   v

Foreword by Dr June Huntington   vii

Preface   xi

Abbreviations   xv

Part One: The Question

1. The terms of the debate   3
   Geoff Meads

2. Realising the potential   9
   Ray Jones

Part Two: The Local Case Material

3. The Cornwall Experience: Locating primary care teams in local community support networks   17
   Murray Cochrane and Derek Law

4. The Hayes Experience: A whole systems approach   25
   Ian Hammond

5. The Bournemouth Experience: Care in the community for elderly people   41
   Diana Churchill and Geoff Colvin

6. The Trowbridge Experience: Care in the community for elderly people   49
   Stephen Henry and Lynn Gaskin

7. The County Durham Experience: From primary health services to primary care teams   61
   Pauline Murray

Part Three: The Response

8. The Communications Challenge: It's good to talk ... and be heard!   75
   Valerie Iles

9. Professional Effectiveness: The Somerset example   87
   Heather Roughton

10. Organisational Effectiveness: The Southampton example   99
    Jill Stannard

11. Managerial Effectiveness: The Wiltshire example   107
    Yvonne Wilkin and Ralph Heywood

12. Personal Effectiveness: Charting icebergs   119
    Andrew Webster

Index   129

Contributors

Diana Churchill
Assistant Public Health Manager, Dorset Health Authority

Murray Cochrane
Director of Development, Cornwall Health Authority

Geoff Colvin
Principal Officer — Health and Disability, Dorset Social Services Department

Lynn Gaskin
Development Worker, Wiltshire Health Authority

Ian Hammond
Chief Executive, Bedford and Shires Health & Care NHS Trust

Stephen Henry
Formerly GP of Lovemead Group Practice, Trowbridge

Ralph Heywood
Principal Officer (Planning and Partnership), Wiltshire County Council

June Huntington
Independent Consultant and Visiting Fellow, King's Fund College, London

Valerie Iles
Director of Health Management Group, City University

Ray Jones
Director of Social Services, Wiltshire County Council

Derek Law
Deputy Director of Social Services, Cornwall County Council

Geoff Meads MA (Oxon) MSc
Professor of Health Services Development, Health Management Group, City University

Pauline Murray
Group Manager, Durham Social Services Department

Heather Roughton
Policy Development Manager, Somerset Social Services Department

Jill Stannard
Commissioning Manager, Commissioning Development, Hampshire Social Services Department

Andrew Webster
Project Director, Joint Reviews of Local Authorities Social Services, The Audit Commission

Yvonne Wilkin
Senior Development Officer (Primary Health Care Services), Wiltshire County Council

Foreword

Just over a year ago I was asked by the NHS Executive to facilitate a two-day workshop entitled *Towards a Primary Care Led NHS: Effective Partnerships for Social Care*. The experience left me feeling like Rip Van Winkle, for I had spent much of the 1970s working with GPs and social workers. Having completed a PhD and published a book about their relationship in 1981, I joined the King's Fund and moved increasingly into management and organisation development in the NHS. Returning to the relationship between the two professions and between their respective organisations 15 years later, I detected little change in their attitude and attributions, in their perceptions of the major problems involved in working more effectively together, and their supposed solutions.

The introduction of a primary care-led NHS, and particularly GP fundholding, aggravated the anxieties of many social workers and their managers. Social Services Departments, like Community Trusts, especially those located in the inner and outer rings of our major cities, have for years had to work with (or as they experience it, *around*) acute variations in the clinical practice of GPs and in the size and structure of their practices.

In some parts of London over 50 per cent of GPs remain single handed, many of them 'disengaged' and 'difficult to access', as described in Chapter 4 of this book. For many residents of these areas, community clinics are their chosen source of primary health care. In these circumstances, 'creative pragmatism', a term used by Wilkin and Heywood in Chapter 11, is the only way forward, and even that must be buttressed by unlimited amounts of what Donald Schon called 'courageous patience'.

Other parts of the country present a different picture, with GPs reaching out to social services, and sharing the hard work but also the exhilaration of combining commitment, expertise, and concern for a population with whom both identify. While, as this book claims, this has in some places been the result of creative and courageous leadership, it has also been the result of the geographically and culturally bounded nature of some towns and villages and the relative stability of a significant proportion of their populations over generations. Health and social care professionals tend to live closer to their work and to relate to each other in roles and settings other than those of work. Those in health authorities and social services departments also tend to stay around for longer than they do in the cities. These communities are also typified by strong traditions of neighbouring and volunteering. While we are aware that some of these 'communities' are changing, and indeed would not attract many of those who by choice live in cities, they do appear to produce far more than their fair share of examples of effective primary health and social care teamwork.

This book explores whether NHS policy changes of the 1990s have created the pre-conditions for a more effective combination of health and social services than was hitherto available. The detailed exploration of this question by Meads and Jones and the subsequent case material will help the new Labour Government decide which of the many health and social care policy initiatives of the past decade should be nurtured and developed and which could usefully be junked.

The book offers a rewarding mix of policy analysis, case material, and reflection. Geoff Meads is an inspired editor, shaping the contributions of authors drawn from a wide variety of professional and organisational settings into a book whose impact is much greater than the sum of its excellent individual chapters. He has a genius for unexpected juxtaposition, evidenced in this collection by the inclusion of remarkable chapters by Valerie Iles and Andrew Webster which remind us of those barriers to effective combination that lie in the psyches of individuals as well as the structures, cultures, and processes of organisations.

The carefully detailed daily realities of the case material and some of the 'Response' chapters of the book reinforce what we have known for a long time: for example, the dependence of 'effective combination' of primary health and social care on good baseline information, agreed as 'good' by all involved; the need to preface combination with flexible, responsive, and sustained practice-based primary care development work; and the need to offer all concerned, managers as well as practitioners, time out to understand each others' worlds.

But there are also revelations, for example the emerging role of nursing, in procuring that more effective combination that is the focus of this book. District Nurses and Health Visitors feature significantly in several of the case studies. There is valuable material here for those working in primary care nursing development. Significantly, the developing role of practice managers does not feature, yet my own work suggests that increasingly the more go-ahead practice managers are initiating and nurturing closer working relationships between their practices and other 'critical partner' organisations in their localities. The other critical player is the Health Authority, whose capacity to change its organisational and managerial spots has been sorely tested by the introduction of a primary care-led NHS. Most have tended so far to concentrate on reconfiguring relationships between primary and secondary care, but their success in so doing depends upon their success in simultaneously reconfiguring the relationship between primary health and social care. The book has much to offer health authority managers as they continue to rethink and reshape their roles.

This is a 'big book': it can't be skimmed or read at a sitting. It demands the undivided attention of its reader. But for those of us who believe that the integration of primary and social care is critical to our capacity to help individuals to *live well* with conditions for which there is no cure, the book will reward the time and attention it deserves to be given.

June Huntington PhD
Independent Consultant and
Visiting Fellow, King's Fund
June 1997

*To my mother,
and brother Colin
— an effective combination*

Preface

During the years I spent as a social work practitioner I became ever more aware of the different, and sometimes contradictory, expectations of those needing and receiving care and those organising its services. From 1980 to 1984 I was a member of a local Social Services Department team in Andover, Hampshire. Caseload management for the team was a part of my responsibilities, which meant that I did a weekly stint as 'Duty Senior' and checked around 50% of the incoming referrals. Although the term 'audit' would then still have been foreign to me or to any of my counterparts, I did as a matter of simple common sense monitor overall trends and do the occasional stocktake to ensure that our workloads were manageable and our patterns of responses broadly consistent.

One such exercise in 1982 I still remember well, not least because it started to trigger the thinking that shapes much of this book. I had become aware that over a period of 6 months or so there had been several self-referrals from female teenagers who had become pregnant. Most were from the dilapidated London overspill estates where both physical and social conditions were in decline and, I think it would be fair to say, at that time, the pastoral care arrangements in the local secondary schools fell some way short of their aspirations. The nearest young mother and baby unit was 30 miles away (a rigorously religious foundation and often full) and abortion remained a controversial issue, not least for some parts of the NHS itself.

It was a situation that warranted enquiry. Social workers had regular liaison arrangements with some GP surgeries, so that it might have been possible to achieve improved collaboration for this particularly vulnerable group of clients. In other cases productive links were less practicable. My assumption was that if we were seeing more pregnant teenagers then this was part of a larger trend. With my suburban middle class conditioning coming through, I fully anticipated that if an adolescent was not telling her parents first that she was pregnant and in need of help, she would go to her doctor. I was completely mistaken. Of the 11 individuals we had seen, only one had actually first made contact with her GP. Even worse, because at least some of my colleagues shared my (false) assumptions, it was evident, on studying the referrals that the expectation that health care support would automatically be forthcoming was frequently colouring our responses to the teenagers themselves. This was too often simply taking the form of one-off advice. We were guilty of crudely categorising pregnancy as 'medical' and therefore an NHS responsibility, whereas in reality, for a variety of reasons, the local social worker in the particular circumstances that applied then in Andover was the first and main port of call for the single pregnant teenager.

The result was that some of these young girls, for a while at least, fell between the statutory health and social services. They sought to enter the system, in effect, by its exit. The service labelling was the wrong way around, and nor was theirs an isolated case. In 1984 when reviewing elderly referrals I found that only one in six of GP referrals (sometimes peremptory one-line demands) for residential care actually warranted, after assessment, an admission to a local authority home. Failure to understand the significance of the service labelling was not simply a public trait; professionals were equally capable of getting it all wrong.

The general need then for a better understanding of health and social services and for their more effective operational links has long been with us. I moved on in 1986 from a social work role to a position in joint planning when the national policy context could scarcely have been more favourable for closer collaboration. *Progress in Partnership* was the banner headline with all sorts of financial and other incentives to 'jointness' on offer in terms of service development, under the auspices of inter-authority member oversight through the statutory District Joint Consultative Committees.

With a few honourable exceptions it simply did not work. Joint developments were limited to the confines of Joint Finance, which was usually underfunded. Far from stimulating a climate of co-operation the culture clash between health authorities protecting their professions and patients, and local authorities representing their committees and clients simply became more overt and more intractable. Long stay hospital closures were clogged up in the mire of disputed cash and capital transfers; such desperately needed new services as domiciliary respite care and drugs misuse counselling became the material for demarcation disputes; and at the macro-level Councillors on the old District Health Authorities fought to gain political control over such groups as adults with learning difficulties and children with physical hardships. The folly of trying even gently to compel local integration through top-down central directives was well and truly exposed.

The present decade has, of course, taken a different course. The advent of the health care internal market, the introduction of performance management, the growth of independent sector social care and more recently the drive towards a primary care-led NHS are creating very different conditions. The question this book explores is whether or not these are preconditions for the more effective combination of health and social services than has hitherto been available. Does the bringing together in general practices of NHS service development, financial control and clinical referral powers, when placed alongside the arrival of local social care managers, mean that the settings of contemporary UK primary care hold the key?

The chapters that follow are written in response to this question. Part One explores *The Question* itself in more detail, setting out the policy framework through which its answers now need to progress. The Director of Wiltshire Social Services, Ray Jones illustrates the potential benefits in prospect in an inspiring piece. Part Two contains a series of local case studies, drawn from districts and counties, from Dorset to Durham, distinguished by a joint leadership commitment to the cause of combining health and social services in primary care. However, this does not mean that they are all success stories. It is, of course, too early to discern established patterns and, amidst the abundant evidence of good practice, there are genuine warning signals too. Both Diana Churchill and Geoff Colvin, and Pauline Murray (Chapters 5 and 7) highlight, for example, the grading anomalies revealed at practice level, particularly between community nurses and social workers once Social Services Department budgets are delegated to the latter in primary care settings. Even in Cornwall, which at this time can truly locate itself at the front end of national developments, the integration of field staff around general practices has not brought budgetary unification and considerable suspicion remains, especially amongst GPs, of 'dumping' as the authorities move to implement their long term Mental Health Services Strategy. The overall message is that of exploring together.

This need to agree on coherent joint processes is reinforced in Part Three which, again drawing on local examples, sets out a framework for co-ordinating development by addressing in harness its personal, organisational, managerial, professional and clinical dimensions. Each one of these is considered separately, with the different strands being drawn together in Valerie Iles' essay (Chapter 8) on the special need for sound management in respect of developments derived from the creative tensions at the interfaces of different agencies and their services. The NHS, in particular, no longer has strategic authorities with the resources and remit to co-ordinate macro-development at a time when the scale and range of change are both unprecedented. The traditional sequence in UK health care of its organisation and managerial structures following the definition of its clinical specialisms and correspondent professions increasingly no longer applies, as the focus on primary care and its consumers leads to more generalist approaches and the emergence of more hybrid health (and social) care organisations. At the same time, paradoxically, as Stephen Henry and Lynn Gaskin point out in Chapter 6, social workers are becoming increasingly specialist as their mandated statutory duties in respect of individual client groups grow. This requires everywhere a generosity of response in terms of participation and shared learning, which is currently exemplified by the willingness in Somerset to pool all sources of data capture and intelligence under the combined heading of 'Evaluation' (Chapter 9). Somerset and its neighbour Wiltshire, we must hope and expect, are the leading examples today for others to follow tomorrow.

Taking the lead always involves risks and exposure, so I am especially grateful to the real mix of contributors to this book for their willingness to stand up and be shot at. The solace is that experience in the present decade suggests that the only place to be is on the pace, for the pace never slackens and those at the back at best get to stay in the pack. For those grappling with the 1997/98 primary care legislative programme the pages that follow will be especially useful. They will soon realise that in policy and practical terms perhaps the main unresolved area for primary care is now the future relationship of its health and social services.

I would like also to thank, in particular, Jane Harding, Pru Daniels and Brenda Wren whose personal contributions have made this book a practical proposition. And finally my gratitude goes to the publisher, Peter Richardson, whose readiness to work together, to take a risk and to set an agenda, captures exactly the key messages of what now follows.

Geoff Meads
Winchester, 7 January 1997

List of Abbreviations

A and E	Accident and Emergency
ADA	Affordable Domestic Assistance
CAB	Citizens Advice Bureau
CCLT	Community Care Liaison Team
CHC	Community Health Council
Cllr	Councillor
CoE	Church of England
CPN	Community Psychiatric Nurse
DHA	District Health Authority
DoH	Department of Health
FE	Further Education
FHSA	Family Health Services Authority
GP	General Practitioner
GPFH	General Practice Fundholding
HHA	Hillingdon Health Authority
JCB	Joint Commissioning Board
JCP	Joint Commissioning Project
LA	Local Authority
LIZ	London Implementation Zone
MA	Medical Audit
MH	Mental Health
MP	Member of Parliament

NHS	National Health Service
NHSE	National Health Service Executive
NVQ	National Vocational Qualification
OT	Occupational Therapist
PCLM	Primary Care Liaison Manager
PCT	Primary Care Team
PHCT	Primary Health Care Team
SSD	Social Services Department
SRB	Single Regeneration Budget
UK	United Kingdom
UPA	Urban Privation Award
VFM	Value for Money
Vol Org	Voluntary Organisation

Part One: The Question

1. Introduction: The terms of the debate

Geoff Meads

WHAT IS THE QUESTION?

The most significant character in the title of this book is its question mark. The papers that follow have, of course, been compiled partly with a view to identifying the opportunities and obstacles that now arise from the advent of a primary care-led NHS,[1] particularly for practitioners at field level in both the health and social services sectors. Their local case material offers much evidence of good practice to learn from and emulate. However, what the papers do not do is seek to supply answers. Together they constitute the fundamental question that policy makers and professionals alike will now have to address over the next few years: is primary care more (or less) effective when health and social services are combined in its settings? This book is designed first and foremost to define and pose this question, and then to begin to determine the agenda required for its response.

It is a question that challenges basic assumptions. Should care as a concept and as a service be regarded as indivisible, or do its different disciplines genuinely and properly reflect the different dimensions of separate human needs? Will the devolution of financial and service planning responsibilities to local levels promote convergence between these disciplines and a broader consensus on public service values; or will devolution result in issues of priority setting becoming the ammunition deployed across a network of local multi-professional battlefields spread throughout the country?

On the answers to these two starter questions alone do the prospects for a future more primary care-centred service system depend. The strategy for the latter has staked out its claims for policy leadership in the contemporary NHS, and beyond, on the basis of a belief in a more holistic philosophy of personal care and a conviction that this, in terms of successful resource management, can be tied to the practical expression of the modern principle of subsidiarity. Failure actually to convert this conviction into practice could all too easily herald a very different direction of travel: polyclinics rather than general practice; institutional outreach facilities in place of community based support; vertical instead of horizontal service integration.

There are, of course, many conservative forces that would favour such a *volte face*. The ranks of medical consultants, long serving NHS general managers, and traditional local authority Labour politicians – to name just three categories at random – include those who are genuinely apprehensive about the consequences of transferring excessive power and responsibility to the multitude of small and medium sized independent sector enterprises that currently occupy the UK primary care sector. And this concern derives from more than just motives of self-preservation variously dressed up as a defence of public accountability. There are democratic issues at stake in terms of a genuine threat to the established role of elected representatives and local government. There are also real risks for the maintenance of professional knowledge and competence in the shift towards a more generic skills mix and flatter team structures that the following case studies suggest the convergence of health and social services in primary care appears inevitably to bring. Above all, however, is the prospect threatened by this convergence: that a policy of combining health and social services in primary care will produce, in the absence of a comprehensive framework for their effective delivery, exactly the opposite impact to that intended: the lowest common denominator as the first point of contact; a new proliferation of next stage specialists but this time in primary care itself; and the determination of resource distribution by local, often commercially oriented objectives, which make a nonsense of both conventional NHS and local authority public service principles and values. In short, the present central rhetoric of 'patient empowerment' and 'client control' would be seen to be just that: ridiculously distant from local realities and discredited as a policy resource for the next century.

Such a Doomsday scenario rings the alarm bells for Community Care itself. Community Care has increasingly been the major policy imperative of the present century. The replacement of long stay institutions, the remarkable growth of voluntary organisations and, in this decade, the establishment of care management principles in practice, each bear witness to a pervasive trend which has shifted assessments of need and the responses required from group norms to individual differences, from collective forms of provision much closer to individual self help. On the back of this trend an open ended Social Security benefits system for residential and nursing home care has been dismantled and limited local authority budgets introduced in its place. The NHS itself has been able to define the local parameters of its medical and continuing care responsibilities, with remarkable consequences for shortened lengths of bed-stays as a result. The shift from collective to personal responsibility has both stimulated and compelled a whole range of new contributions, not least financial. Co-payments and Community Care have rapidly become a combined course in the 1990s. Which is the appropriate point at which to return to primary care. Primary health services have always played an important part in Community Care. But until the present decade this was clearly one discrete contribution, amongst several, with definite limitations. Primary care-led purchasing has changed all that. GP Fundholding, in particular, as it has expanded to encompass the commissioning of Community Health Services, has completely altered the rules of the game. With social care management following in its wake, leading edge general practices now term themselves 'Community Care Centres'[2] and the boundaries between primary and community care become increasingly hard to discern.

The Family Health Services at the heart of UK primary care rely, of course, on various types of co-payments not just for their present survival but for their future expansion. The levels of prescription charges, dental treatment payments and eye test fees are essential factors in business viability. The potential fusion of primary and community care signifies a mixed economy of both care purchasers and providers in which the private or public status of a local agency may well seem to be of increasing irrelevance. The wider implications of such a development can scarcely be underestimated. The perspective becomes that in which the agents of expanded primary health, probably unwittingly, become the vehicles through which not simply the practice of Community Care is effected but the relationship between the State and the individual citizen significantly changed.

THE question that therefore emerges from combining, let us assume effectively, health and social services in primary care is quite simply, '*Who will pay the price?*'

WHAT IS THE ARGUMENT?

The argument is essentially twofold. Are the forces for the convergence of health and social services now more compelling than those, both old and sometimes new, which operate to keep them apart? And if the former are in the ascendancy, does this signify a combination of better all-round effectiveness or not? We should not automatically assume that a positive answer to the first question automatically leads to a 'yes' response to the second. Cause and correlation are quite different.

The traditional reasons for divergence have, of course, been endlessly repeated, being usually expressed in terms of the differences between the two 'lead' professionals: the social worker and the GP. June Huntington's classic analysis in 1981 of the inter-occupational relationship has, in many ways unfortunately, stood the test of time remarkably well.[3] The relational orientations have often remained quite different. The psycho-systems language of social work remains as much a barrier as medical terminology and the fundamental gap in status. The GP conventionally brings hierarchial expectations to proposals for collaboration, while egalitarian values are at the heart of social work practice. Inter-professional primary care can still all too readily seem a distant dream.

But this is now too pessimistic. Many of the reasons given by Huntington for divergence are no longer quite so persuasive. The age gap has reduced; GPs are now not so characteristically male and social workers female. In 1996 50% of the former's recruits were women. The split between psycho-social and bio-medical care is not so pronounced, as both Social Services Departments and General Practices have in this decade had to respond to national policies for care in the community and health promotion which have literally put an added premium on general preventive and maintenance services. Even the impact of contrasting employment status seems to be diminishing. The 1997 Primary Care Act appears to be ushering in a new era of contractual and organisational flexibility in which, for example, salaried status may in many places apply as much to primary care physicians as it does to nurse practitioners or social workers.

Such developments suggest that the forces for convergence now stand a better chance. These are summarised in Box 1.1 and taken together constitute a powerful case for progress. When such principles as care management emerge out of reciprocal self-interest there is, of course, always a better prospect of their successful conversion into practice.

Box 1.1 Health and social services in primary care — the forces for convergence

1. New legislative levers	— for example, GPFH purchasing of Community Health Services, Social Services care management requirement for GP contribution to individual needs assessment.
2. New financial structures	— for example, devolved NHS budgetary control to practice level alongside locality care management allocations, with equivalent downward pressures.
3. New organisational developments	— for example, new NHS regulations releasing HCHS capital to primary care with organisational status that can now attract local authority grants and funding.
4. New professional flexibility	— for example, via NVQ and range of new para-medical qualifications leading to revised skills mix and substitution of specialists by generic care workers in both health and social services.
5. New public accountability frameworks	— arising from the new consumerism, recognising that elected or professional representative structures are no longer enough and that, with the new range of direct financial and service responsibilities, popular support for local priority setting must be demonstrable by all players in the extended primary care setting.

The convergence of health and social services in primary care continues to contain real risks, however persuasive its case has now become. The theory and practice of social care and its values — acceptance, self-determination, solidarity — are still much less well established than those of clinicians. The danger of merger becoming take-over is there, and, some would argue, even more pronounced now that entrepreneurial GPs are released from the shackles of an organisational form that compelled them to be in partnership with each other. There is no realistic prospect of local GP commissioning groups ever becoming Primary Care Sub-Committees of the local authority. All history and culture argues against this. The convergence of health and social services in primary care is coming but central policies which pave the way for genuinely holistic care must not be translated locally into the totalitarian tyranny of tomorrow's GPs.

WHAT IS THE ANSWER?

Where does all this leave the argument on the second, more significant question posed at the start of the preceding section: 'If the forces for the convergence of health and social services are now more compelling does this point to a combination of better all-round effectiveness or not?' Will primary care provide the answer?

The response, at this stage, has to be annoyingly evasive. As many of the chapters that follow will illustrate, the persuasive answers are still those that focus on process, not outcomes. Certainly, the case for the shift from individually oriented primary health services to effective population based primary care can be backed up by, for example, illustrations of new data exchanges, practice accreditation and similar organisational systems for better collaboration. But equally, the case for decline can be made just as powerfully through pointing to the lack of grassroots motivation, the absence of real performance management to make *It* happen, the growing need to retain genuine specialisms (e.g. in mental health), and above all the dearth of co-ordinated development programmes which address effectiveness in all its dimensions: professional/clinical, organisational, managerial and personal.

The answer then is to go cautiously in order to become credible. Locating effective combinations of health and social services in primary care is an exploration. What we can be sure of now, however, is that this is an exploration we have no option but to undertake.

REFERENCES

1. The policy banner of a 'Primary Care-Led NHS' emerged in the NHSE's national communication on 'Developing NHS Purchasing and GP Fundholding' EL(94) 79 in October 1994, after which a series of central policy documents culminated in the Secretary of State for Health's White Papers 'Choice and Opportunity' and 'Delivering the Future' issued by the Department of Health in October and December 1996 respectively to preface the government's 1997 Primary Care Bill.
2. Refer, for example, to Robinson B 1994 Integrating Health and Social Care: The Lyme Community Care Unit, Community Care Management and Planning 2(5): pp 139–143, and Pietroni P 1995 The Integrated Community Care Practice In Meads G (ed) Future Options for General Practice. Radcliffe Medical Press, Oxford, pp 133–148
3. Huntington J 1981 Social Work and General Medical Practice: Collaboration or Conflict. Allen and Unwin, London, pp 155–173

2. Realising the potential[1]

Ray Jones

Wiltshire is the leading exponent of combining health and social services in the UK. Its leadership is best placed accordingly to set out our future agenda. Ray Jones is Director of Wiltshire Social Services.

THE ISSUES

The drive within health care policy to develop a Primary Care-Led NHS has been especially promoted by encouraging General Practitioner Fundholding (GPFH). There is no doubt that those GPs who have championed fundholding are succeeding in delivering a wider range of services locally and in developing GP practices which are much more consumer-friendly. They have drawn into their practice settings a wider range of health staff to provide a more integrated, one-stop shop local health service. They have also taken forward the message that health promotion is as important as treating illness with a range of health promotion and monitoring services now available from the GP practice. Add to these gains the focus on performance and efficiency, and the increasing use of purchasing power being achieved by many GP fundholding practices, and it is easy to understand why there seems to be increasing mileage in a Primary Care-Led NHS.

The description above, however, relates entirely to health care services. There is now a greater potential for primary care which stretches beyond the health service. The primary care setting also provides an opportunity to develop more locally accessible and responsive social care as well as health services. This will help to breach the boundary between health care and social care services (as provided by local authority social services), enhancing again the opportunity for a one-stop shop health and social care access point, generating the potential gains of having integrated health and social care budgets to avoid accusations of, and attempts at, cost shunting, and would also promote more integrated and strategic planning of services for local populations.

In addition, it could provide within one setting a further enhancement to the skills mix available to the local population, with the potential for social workers and local authority occupational therapists to be working as members of the primary care team. It also could generate greater efficiency with other non-social services members of the primary care team being given the opportunity to act as 'accredited care managers'. They would participate in the local authority's training for its care management staff, and then be able to spend directly against social services budgets in arranging, for example, home care, day care or respite care services without the delay and duplication of having to request a new and further assessment from a social services social worker or an occupational therapist.

If there is greater potential for a Primary Care-Led NHS than just thinking about improved local health care services, then what might prevent these benefits being realised? What also might limit the further promotion of a Primary Care-Led NHS as a future model for health care provision?

PRESENT PROBLEMS

There are a number of difficulties with the current concept of a Primary Care-Led NHS which limit its potential:

1. Those GPs who have actively embraced fundholding are not necessarily representative of most GPs. There are GPs reluctant to embrace fundholding, and the additional responsibilities it entails, and there will be some practices where others would be very anxious about them taking the budgetary control responsibilities that go along with fundholding.
2. The GP champions of fundholding, and those who are promoting a Primary Care-Led NHS, are likely to be those with drive, imagination and considerable commitment. General practice across the country is very disparate, with wide variations in standards and in performance. This is bound to limit how much responsibility, overall, can be passed to a GP. There must be limitations on the responsibilities and opportunities than can be passed to those whose competence may be more limited or whose behaviour might be somewhat maverick and, indeed, possibly eccentric!

3. Some GPs are also now reflecting on being tied into business partnerships which restrict their mobility; and this may be a particular issue where GPs wish to work part-time, take career breaks, or want to be geographically mobile. Salaried status should now assist many of these aspirations.
4. Whilst GPs are not salaried employees of the health service but are independent contractors, there must be concern about how much public funding can be placed within the direct spend control of GPs. We are no longer talking about relatively small sums of money. Practices are beginning to control budgets of six figures and beyond. If the relevant practice population social care expenditure was also allocated to a GP-controlled (and, indeed in some ways,-owned) primary care setting, then GPs, as independent, self-employed operators, would be responsible for potentially millions of pounds of public funding. There must be limits to what degree of responsibility, and what amounts of public money, can be handed to GPs as independent practitioners.

   There is also disquiet that GPs, as small business persons, may lack accountability in deploying large amounts of public funding, and it would not take many scandals, about the possible misuse or misdirection of this funding by some GPs to undermine public confidence in fundholding.
5. There is also concern, and this is expressed by many GPs themselves, about the amount of organisational and management time required from them. This detracts from the best deployment of the scarce resource they provide in terms of clinical expertise and is in danger of increasingly removing them from patient care.
6. The training of clinicians does not best prepare GPs, overall, to be well-developed resource and personnel managers, team players and developers. Some GPs clearly have these skills, and some GPs very much wish to be able to have these responsibilities as a part of their working week. Indeed, some GPs may wish to move away from the clinical practice to develop the much more managerial and strategic roles that might be offered within a large fundholding practice, but this is not the position for all, or necessarily most, GPs.
7. There is public disquiet about GP fundholding, and a concern on the part of patients, that decisions will be taken not on the basis of clinical assessment and need but on the basis of budget availability. There is no escaping the rationing and gatekeeping

role which has been, and will need to be played by GPs, but GPs have also had a role as advocates for their patients. Giving GPs the ultimate frontline budget responsibility has led to comments that their recommendations are determined by 'not what's best for the patient' but 'what's best for the budget'.

A POSSIBLE WAY FORWARD

Recognising the comments above about the potential gains of a Primary Care-Led NHS, with the increased integration of social care services within the primary care setting, but also noting the potential difficulties of having a Primary Care-Led NHS driven forward by GPs and the fundholding concept, does require that other models are considered. Some of these will need to challenge potential vested interests and power structures and therefore, it is recognised that they may not be easily grasped politically.

But, while there is still a debate about, for example, the separation or integration of health and social care services, the role of central government and of local authorities, and the purchaser/provider separation within the health service, it is timely to reflect on other possible models.

One possible model would be to continue to develop the primary care setting, to look towards an increased integration of social care alongside health care services within the primary care setting, but to recognise that this does increase the organisational and managerial load within the primary care setting. Larger multidisciplinary primary care teams, with increasing budget responsibility and purchasing power, will require strong resource and personnel management. They will also require that the clinical skills and time of GPs are not over consumed in the requirement to become business managers. As noted above, GPs may not have the interest, experience or skills to take on this enhanced and increasing business management role with greater resource responsibilities.

This would suggest, therefore, the requirement that primary care continues to be developed as a locally accessible, acceptable, responsive and integrated service, but with the role of the GP primarily recognised as that of clinician within the enhanced primary care team. There is a general management role within primary care and it should not be assumed that this necessarily falls to the GP. Indeed, although some GPs will fulfil this role very successfully and will want to take on this responsibility and to move away from clinical practice, the role should be shaped separately from the clinical role and should be recruited to appropriately, drawing on those with relevant experience and skills.

This challenges the concept of primary care as GP-owned and GP-driven. However, it does offer the opportunity of improving management within primary care, of building primary care back into a stronger accountable public service framework, and it also provides the potential of integrating primary care and services which are currently the separate responsibility of Community Health Services trusts. It would be possible to look towards Community Health Services Trusts and General Practices moving closer to organisational integration, rather than having the unsatisfactory power plays that currently exist between the provision of community services within primary care and the continued attempts by NHS Trusts to be the prevalent providers and shapers of community services.

THE CHALLENGE

The statements above are based on a commitment that primary care should be a major driving force for the NHS both in shaping services and in providing services. More integrated local provision crossing the health and social care divide will be welcomed and will generate gains for local people. However, this does require a recasting of the concept of primary care away from GP small businesses to a stronger focus on well-managed, large-scale primary care teams and on budgets which are linked into a publicly recognised and accepted system of accountability back through the democratic structures in general government and within local government. It provides the scope for greater permeability (influence by local people) about the shape of services, greater accountability, and greater legitimacy. It is an opportunity not to be lost.

REFERENCE

1. This chapter is based upon Jones R 1996 Realizing the Potential. Primary Care Management 6(7/8): pp 37–39

Part Two: The Local Case Material

3. The Cornwall Experience: Locating primary care teams in local community support networks

Murray Cochrane and Derek Law

Cornwall has traditionally seen itself as off the map, and off the pace in terms of pioneering service developments. With recent changes in the senior management of both the new Health Authority and the Social Services Department, and the emergence of a particularly creative set of GP purchasers, this image is now rapidly changing. The authors, Murray Cochrane and Derek Law, are at the forefront of these changes and nowhere is field social work so well established with general practice as in Cornwall. This chapter highlights in particular the increased focus on prevention and self-help that can emerge from these new partnerships but with the separate budgetary structures remaining firmly in force, the message is that such partnerships should still be based on respect for separate professional contributions rather than a full fusion. Cornwall geographically and now also figuratively can genuinely view itself as the starting point for the UK health and social care system.

CARE MANAGEMENT MEANS IN CORNWALL

The phone rings in the local Social Services office:

'Good morning, Social Services Department, how can I help you?'

'Oh, hello there, my mother, Mrs P., who is 74, needs some help from Social Services.'

'O.K.' says the Receptionist, 'Could you tell me your mother's name and address please, and then the name and address of her General Practitioner?'

There then follows a short discussion on the needs of the caller's mother as perceived by her and her son, and the referral is processed straight through to the Case Co-ordinator for that patch who, because the presenting needs were perceived as non-complex, arranges an assessment and package to be in place within 3 days.

The second question asked of the son, that is the name and address of his mother's GP, lies at the very heart of the Cornish system for Community Care, which recognises the importance of the links between social services and primary care in local community support networks.

So what is the Cornwall Care Management System? Care Management can mean different things to different Authorities, but quite often care managers are qualified social workers or occupational therapists who provide assessments and services for people with complex needs or where there is likely to be a major life change, such as admission to residential or nursing home care.

What was different in Cornwall from the outset, however, was that the arrangements should centre importantly on providing services quickly to people with less complex problems, recognising that these clients were often more than able to determine their own needs without time consuming and sometimes expensive professional guidance.

In thinking through the 'assessment of need' aspect of the Cornish system, the Social Services Department was helped in its deliberations by some important local research undertaken by the Social Services Inspectorate in 1991 by David Raw and Colin Shipley.[1] Their study of referrals and services in the Penwith District of Cornwall showed that most people with less complex needs knew largely what they required themselves and gained little or nothing from the interventions of a range of expensive professionals, like district nurses, occupational therapists and social workers simply to confirm what they were asking for. The other conclusion from the research was that many people needed only the minimum of services and interventions to continue to live in their own homes or independently, and that early and rapid interventions were likely to sustain the individual's self-confidence and feelings of independence.

The other interesting feature from the study was that it was estimated that 80% of the cases relating to the needs of elderly or physically disabled people were of a less complex or non-complex nature, which appeared to be a message about the levels of skills required in carrying out assessments and delivering packages of care.

Cornwall Case Co-Ordinators

Following the Penwith study, and in preparation for Community Care, Cornwall Social Services initiated two pilot projects in different areas of the county when it tested a model which targeted its most experienced and qualified workers on the anticipated 20% of complex cases. On the other hand, the 80% non-or less complex high volume cases of older people and those with a disability were processed through a more practical and appropriately trained workforce.

A new type of worker created through this process, which was eventually implemented fully in April 1993, was that of Case Co-ordinator. Many of the staff came from posts such as social work assistants, senior home helps, occupational therapy assistants or had auxiliary nurse background. Now trained to NVQ Level III in Social Care, some 65 Case Co-ordinators were initially recruited, each linked to one or more of the 80 GP practices located in the county.

This brings us back to the Social Services Department Receptionist's second question to the son of Mrs P., that is the name of the GP. This question immediately elicits the basic information required to identify the name of the Case Co-ordinator who would deal with the case so that clients and all professional and other social and health care colleagues are aware of the named Co-ordinator in any given case. This notion is based on the assumption that the great majority of us have a GP with whom we are registered and evidence from the Penwith and other studies has shown that the General Practice is the favoured place for older people to go when in need of information and advice.

GPs and other health professionals have seen it as an important feature of recognising the links between primary care and community care and, although it has not been possible to achieve a physical location in GP surgeries for all Case Co-ordinators, a great majority are out there in the community, either in surgeries, church halls, residential homes or other such local venues. This achieved the objective of locating Case Co-ordinators as close to the local community they serve as possible, particularly important for people in Cornwall who suffer from a general lack of accessibility to services because of rural scatter.

While out on their local visits to clients Case Co-ordinators make use of laptop computers immediately to tap in the identified needs of the people they have assessed which are then transferred through modems to the seven local district offices where this core assessment is then processed to ensure delivery of a package of services to the client's home within a 3-day period. This process not only ensures a speedy response but also provides a less bureaucratic system by inputting assessment information straight through to a central ordering system which cuts out unnecessary paperwork.

With regard to complex cases, the Case Co-ordinators have been trained to recognise when an individual has complex needs or, indeed, when they are out of their depth. Such cases are referred to the managers of the system, that is Cornwall's version of care managers who are not only responsible for Case Co-ordinators, but also for a range of professionals. Each of the 21 care managers supervises between three and five Case Co-ordinators together with a number of social workers, occupational therapists and technicians.

In complex cases the care manager commissions a specialist worker, usually a social worker or occupational therapist, to undertake an assessment for which a package is guaranteed to be in place for the client within a 28-day period. Any urgent cases, whether non-complex or complex, are guaranteed some form of package on the same day.

Cornwall's structure is described in Figure 3.1

Cornwall's Care Management model has now been in place for over 3 years and the case profile has levelled out to around about 70% non-complex and 30% complex, with the division of referrals for Case Co-ordinators and social workers or occupational therapists reflecting this division almost precisely. Certainly, in terms of volume of referrals, the numbers went far beyond those expected from original calculations. In 1994 approximately 33 000 referrals were made to the Care Management System from which 24 000 care packages were arranged. Of these over 80% were delivered within 5 working days of the referral and there is little doubt that, without the current system wherein appropriate skills and resources have been deployed to appropriate levels of need, there would be waiting lists for people with less complex needs while assessments were undertaken by specialist workers, who would undoubtedly have had to concentrate on the higher priority complex work.

Apart from the obvious achievement of getting packages in place within 3 days for non-complex and 28 days for complex cases, the Cornwall Care Management System also empowers clients by enabling them to express and clearly determine their needs and, in large part, have them met very speedily through the Case Co-ordinator. Responsibility is also devolved to Case Co-ordinators who are

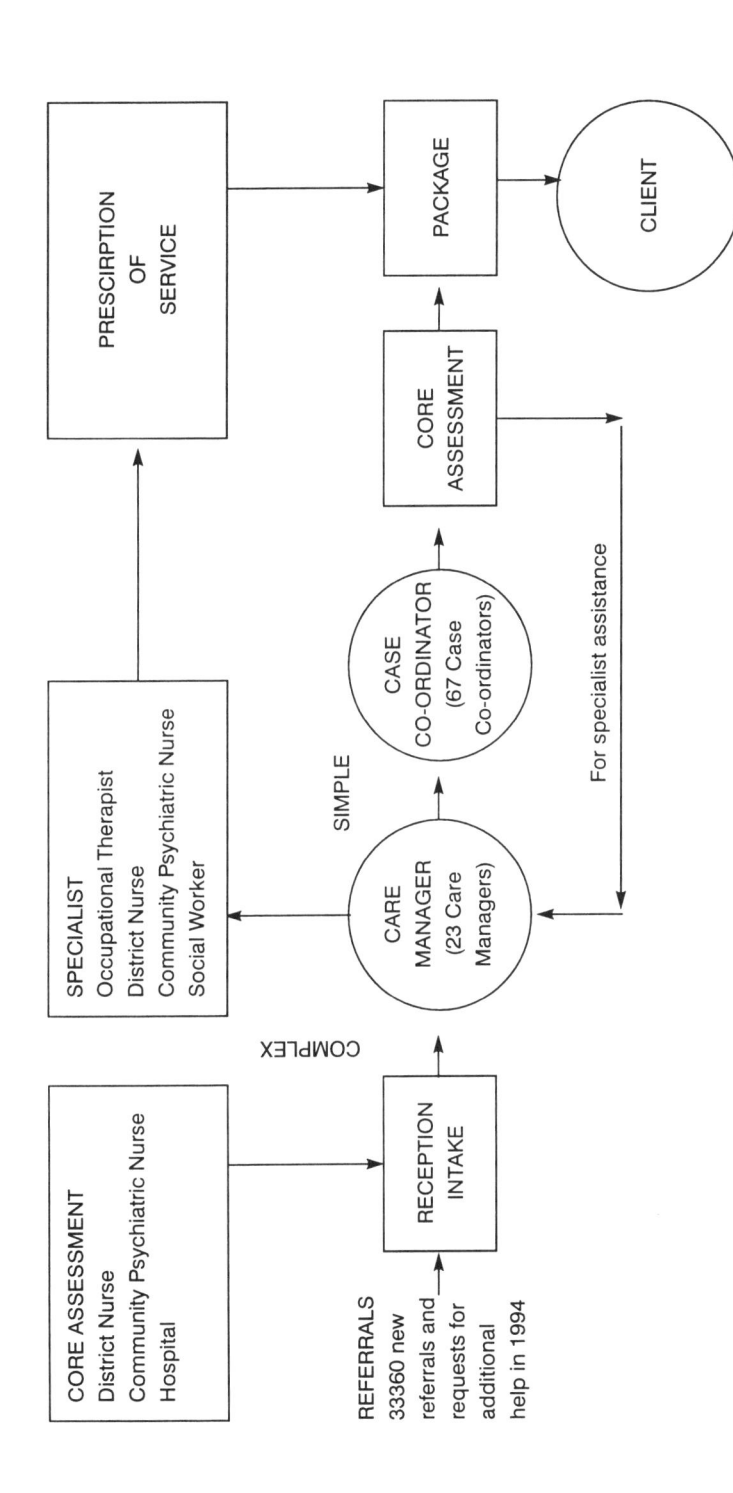

Fig. 3.1 Cornwall's care management model

empowered to make straightforward decisions on care packages in the majority of cases. Although the 65 Case Co-ordinators do not control the spend, they will actually be committing an average of £100 000 each on care packages throughout 1996/97. Working the Care Management System together and largely in partnership with primary care health colleagues, such as GPs, district nurses and auxiliary staff of the local Community Trust has led to good grass roots communications, particularly between health and social services staff.

The general view is that there has been an intervention in a preventive way early enough in an older or physically disabled person's life to maximise their potential for remaining independent and in their own home for as long as possible. Reviews are undertaken by Case Co-ordinators either 6-monthly or when the client needs change. Clearly all primary care workers involved in a particular locality are partners in this process, reinforcing the importance of the joint team operating as an important local support network.

Indeed, the Cornwall Care Management System has been reviewed formally twice since its introduction and the role of Case Co-ordinator in particular and the system generally has been praised by Cornwall's GPs and other health staff. It is seen as a system which gets essential services to people with a minimum of intervention and a maximum involvement of the clients patients themselves.

THE PRIMARY CARE PERSPECTIVE

From the perspective of primary health care, this experience of community care has highlighted some simple yet powerful themes. Taking as an example one of the GP practices in North Cornwall, an 'away weekend' was the starting point for a team development initiative which included the local Social Services staff. It was a traumatic experience but with spin-offs which dramatically affected the practice's style of working. The key factors identified as important for care in the community to work at practice level were:

- good 'grass-roots' communications;
- a clear identity of responsible individuals (who's who);
- a local budget allocation; and
- a listening approach to show that people across organisational divides really are working together and acknowledging each other's needs.

The care management system described earlier has been shown to achieve the practice's objectives. The expected case breakdown has been borne out by the workload generated from the practice population. Both simple cases (such as the need for a walking stick) and specialised needs (such as those of the deaf) have been met within the target timescales of 3 days and 28 days respectively.

Drawing out the lessons from the GPs' experience, it is evident that empowerment of both patients and the Case Co-ordinators is a key to success. This has been coupled with devolution to Case Co-ordinators of budgetary responsibility for simple solutions. For practice staff, the health and social care interface is all about day-to-day communication, not the politics of paranoia. In short, people on the ground have been able to deliver fast, practical results, get on well together and keep within budget, while the large organisations deal with the complex policy issues associated with eligibility criteria for health services. Interestingly, the two ways forward highlighted as necessary by practice staff in the light of their experience are:

- more personal involvement by General Practitioners in relating to the wider team of practice-based professionals; and
- keeping separate budgets for health and social services. This is regarded as the most straightforward way to manage services by that particular practice. Operational staff were quite comfortable with working out who should cover the costs of particular patient needs.

Clearly, there is a range of opinion about many of the issues associated with linking health and social care at practice-level. However, the experience in Cornwall demonstrates that practical solutions based on well-founded research are within our grasp.

REFERENCE

1. Raw D, Shipley C A 1991
   Study of Referrals and Services provided in the Penwith District of Cornwall. A Social Services' Inspectorate report

4. The Hayes Experience: A whole systems approach

Ian Hammond

Political differences, both between and within health and more particularly local authorities, are usually cited as the major reason why greater progress has not been made in the past on health and social services collaboration. As Ian Hammond, the former local NHS Director of Commissioning, so vividly describes in the pages that follow, nowhere has this been more true than on the outskirts of London in Hillingdon. Nowhere, as a result, given the hard pressures on resources and escalating needs levels, has a robust strategic approach been more required. Ian's is an immensely encouraging account of how such an approach, if well managed, can not only involve primary care but successfully address its future development as an integral part of a local community's wider public service requirements. Drawing directly on the lessons of major acute sector reconfiguration reviews, the Hayes Health Plan is also an example of how all players can be brought together to share information, intelligence and concerns and to support each other in planning a much more broad based approach to primary care than the past preoccupation with separate professional and organisational boundaries would ever permit.

This chapter describes the genesis of a joint approach that looked at the health and associated needs of a local population in part of the London Borough of Hillingdon, created multi-agency partnerships around key principles, and considered options for the provision of primary care in its widest sense, including social services. The 'Hayes Health Plan' is currently out for discussion. Its status is more 'Green Paper' than 'White Paper'. The project leaves the situation open to exploiting new freedoms outlined in the government's Primary Care White Papers *'Choice and Opportunity'* and *'Delivering the Future'*,[1] most of which seem likely to endure the change of Government in 1997.

An analysis of what has so far worked and what has not is also given. Like all good soap operas, the plot in Hayes is complex and continuing. It is sufficiently familiar to be reassuring yet sufficiently unpredictable to hold one's interest. And we do not know the ending yet though we will have very considerable influence over it! Now read on ...

THE HILLINGDON CONTEXT

To appreciate properly the influences behind our approach, it is worth sketching in the key characteristics of Hillingdon, its health and social services infrastructure.

Hillingdon is the third largest and western most London Borough. It has one of the smallest Health Authority populations at about 250 000 and enjoys the advantage of being coterminous with a single Local Authority. The District Health Authority and FHSA were managed together since 1993 and cohabited for 18 months before formal merger from April 1996 with an almost entirely new Board. A number of factors make life more complex. There are four NHS trusts in Hillingdon and in 1994 two of them (Mount Vernon Hospital and Hillingdon Community Trust) merged with partners across separate boundaries. It also has 50 million passengers passing through Heathrow, a fact which affects demand for both health and social services. On the edge of the conurbation there are also a number of other cross-boundary flows: in particular, up to 10% of Hillingdon residents have a non-Hillingdon GP.

Just over half the population has a fundholding GP and there is in 1997 a Total Purchasing Pilot scheme covering 20 000 patients in the north of the Borough. A locality commissioning approach has been adopted.

Within the Local Authority there have been significant changes over the last few years. In 1993 overall control passed from Conservative to Labour with a majority of one after a bye-election. At the last local elections Labour control was consolidated. The Chair of Social Services has changed four times over the last 4 years, as has the Director. Under the last Conservative administration Social Services and Education were briefly merged. There is therefore a history of significant and frequent change of structures and of senior personnel in both Health and Social Services organisations.

The Local Authority expresses a keen interest in health, particularly under the aegis of its Anti-Poverty Programme. A number of joint initiatives aimed at health improvement in the context of community development have been put together.

A bit about Hayes

You have probably been to or through Hayes, but you may not have noticed. It consists of eight electoral wards in the South Eastern quadrant of Hillingdon. Hayes is sandwiched between the A40 and Heathrow Airport, with Ealing to the East and Uxbridge and West Drayton to the West. It is bisected by the main Paddington line and the M4. There are several other major roads which facilitate transport but serve as physical barriers for local populations and need to be taken into account in planning services (Fig. 4.1).

Since the 1970s, the traditional manufacturing industries have been in decline and there are large tracts of derelict land and buildings. More recently the development of the high-tech Stockley Business Park and the provision of service industries associated with Heathrow have brought new types of work. The Local Authority was successful in its Single Regeneration Budget (SRB) bid which aims to secure £80m investment into the Hayes/West Drayton corridor, 20% of which would come from a public sector consortium, including the NHS. There are also plans for a fifth terminal at Heathrow (T5) which, if successful, would have a profound impact on the population, economy and geography of Hayes.

The analogy of a family tree is useful for describing the genesis of a joint strategic approach to primary care in Hayes (Fig. 4.2).

Demography and epidemiology

The population of 72 500 is younger but poorer than the other localities in Hillingdon. It has higher proportions of people in socio-economic classes IV and V; more single parent families; more unemployment and overcrowding than elsewhere. It also has the highest proportion of residents from a minority ethnic population at 22%, mostly of Indian origin. There are growing numbers of refugees, especially from Somalia.

Unsurprisingly, the averages for the locality mask pockets of significant deprivation and relative affluence within Hayes.

The established link between poverty and ill health is evident in Hayes where its demography is reflected in higher levels of ill health

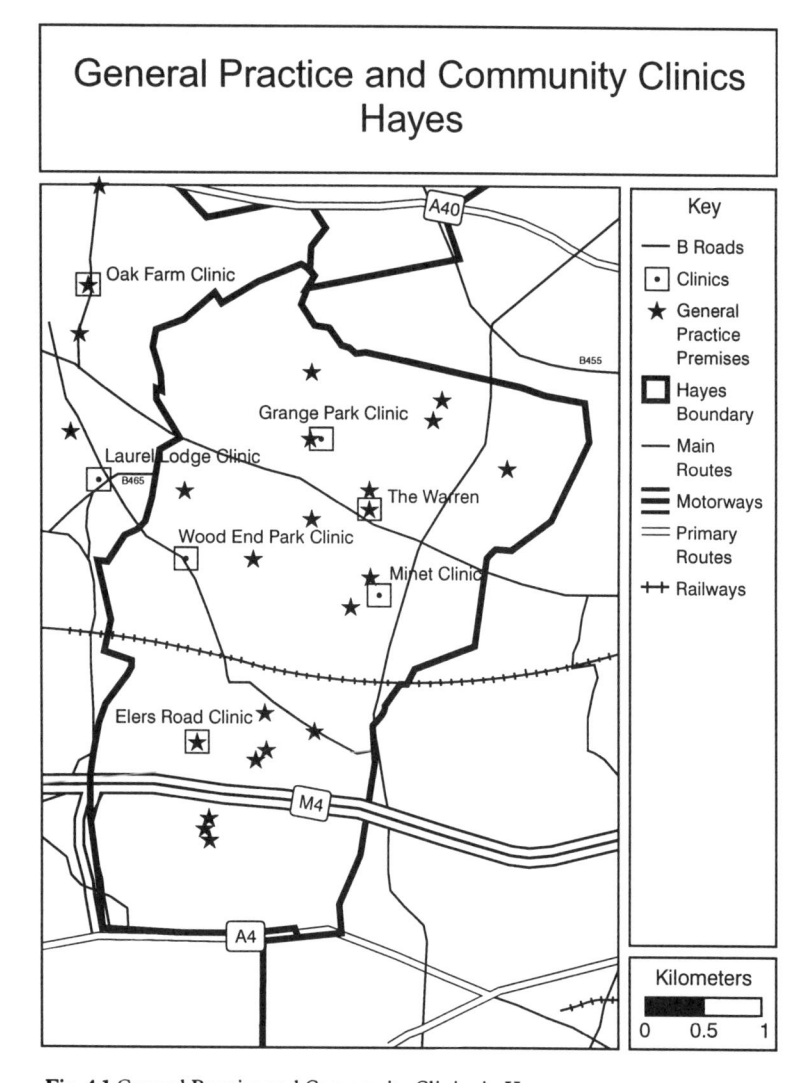

Fig. 4.1 General Practice and Community Clinics in Hayes

and demand for healthcare than elsewhere in Hillingdon. Despite its relatively young population Hayes has a higher proportion of people with a long-term illness and the Standardised Mortality Ratios for seven of the eight electoral wards are above the England average, three of them significantly so. Mental Health admissions reflecting the burden of psychiatric morbidity are also above average.

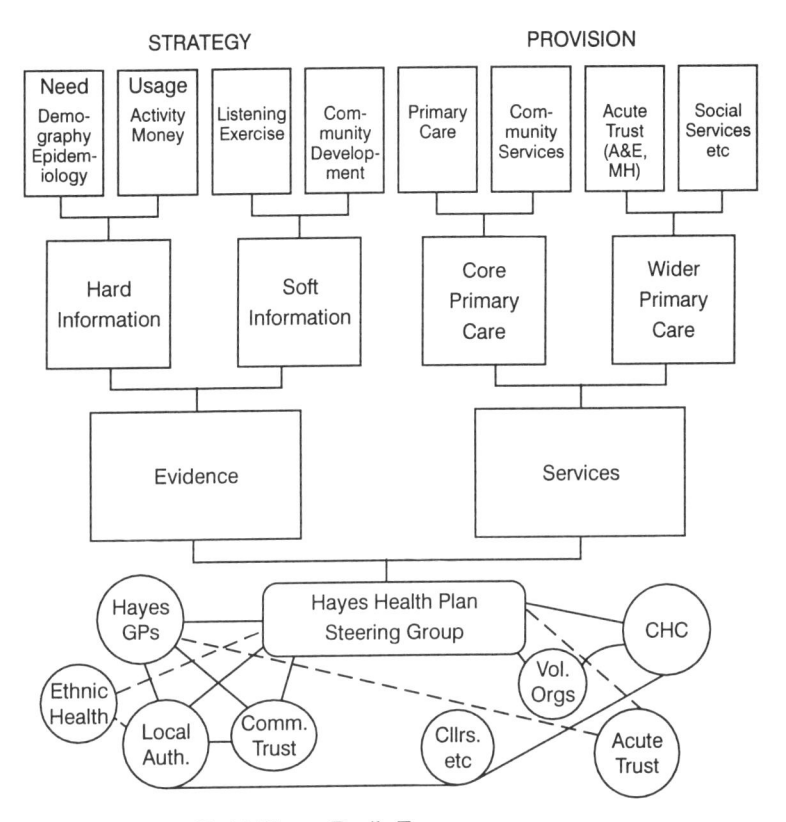

Fig. 4.2 The Hayes Health Plan — Family Tree

RESOURCE USAGE

Clearly any strategic review of service provision needs to identify what services are available, the extent to which they are used (appropriately or otherwise); and what they cost. Whilst such information ought to be readily available often it is not. And even if it is available, it is not necessarily comprehensive or reliable. However, it is important to use the material we have and check out its veracity by engaging with a wide range of providers and users. Despite increased levels of ill health the uptake of such services as dentistry, immunisation, cervical screening and the provision of preventive services such as asthma and diabetic clinics in general practice is lower than average.

The Health Authority is committed to the principle of equity of access based on need. Because budgets for health services are constrained (Hayes is outside the London Implementation Zone [LIZ]) any investment must come from within the Health Authority's total resource. This implies transferring resources from more affluent areas where health need is less and services are superior to many available in Hayes. It is easy to assume because levels of ill health are higher and uptake of services is low, that the cost is less. This is not necessarily so, particularly if the local population are referred by their GPs more to secondary care, or they elect to use community clinics and/or Accident and Emergency Departments in preference to primary care, as some evidence would suggest. There may well be scope for savings in secondary and/or community services by providing higher quality primary care. It is therefore critical to scope resource use for the whole borough to identify sources of investment. But it does not stop there. One persistent strand in the Hayes Health Plan is the need to look at publicly funded resources across the board and identify opportunities to reduce duplication of effort and premises and to look at opportunities for joint provision of services as well as their joint commissioning.

Within the Health Authority, a major exercise to identify resource usage across the board was mounted as part of a wider locality based approach. It will have benefits for the distribution of resources based on need to the other two localities. Discussions of a collaborative nature based on Hayes have been held at Board level with the Local Authority, including the Directors of Education, Housing and Local Services as well as Social Services, and these continue. Strategic agreement has also been reached on the sharing of key information on an electoral ward basis. An example for Townfield ward in central Hayes is set out in Box 4.1.

Hard information for planning purposes involved a number of disciplines within the Health Authority, including Public Health, Finance and Information and Commissioning. It is increasingly shared with other key agencies. But the hard information only comes to life when it links with softer sources of information. Our 'listening exercise' approach, associated with consultation on macro level strategic change combined with a community development approach, empowered local communities to achieve a small scale but meaningful and practical change for the better. We called it the Hayes Listening Exercise.

THE HAYES LISTENING EXERCISE

Just like any family tree, the structure described is highly simplified

Box 4.1 Townfield ward profile

Population 1991

All ages	Male	Female	Total	Projection 2001	% change 1991–2001
	11 003	5585	16 588	17 325	4.4%

Double amount of males to females. A significant increase in 20–39 age group in both male and female. Fewer in their 60s and 70s

Standardised Mortality Ratios 1988–92
All ages   106.67   A very high ranking, 6th out of 29

Children
Under 5s   796   Projected 9.0% increase by year 2001
Schools: Dr Triplett's C of E Junior and Infant School, Minet Junior School, Minet Infant School, Hayes Centre College of FE

Elderly
1991 Over 60s 1999 (18.2% of ward population) HHA total = 19.5%
Pensioners alone: 572 (76.3% female)

Registered Small Homes: 49 Cranbourne Way (3 persons with mental health problems), 51 Cranbourne Way (3 persons with mental health problems), Quenchwell Rest Home (12 elderly people)
Residential Care Homes: 4 and 6 Precinct Road (5 adults with learning disabilities), 36 and 38 Yeading Lane (6 adults with learning disabilities)
Nursing Homes: Hayes Cottage Nursing Home (elderly over 60, short stay, convalescent, mildly confused)

Long Standing Illness
1361: 12.4% (HHA average 9.9%)

Deprivation Factors
4048 Households   Jarman UPA + 18.98 (1981: +3.55)

	Ethnicity	Unemployment	Unskilled	No CH	LA Housing
%	24.2	10.3	5.1	10.3	28.6
HHA Average	12.3	6.8	4.3	11.4	15.7

Ethnicity is high, particularly Indian, being 14.4% of the ward population

Primary and Community Care
GPs:
— Drs Ruparelia, Sethi & Sethi, 1 Fulwood Close (GPFH/6th Wave SF)
— Dr Goud, 'Kincora', Coldharbour Lane
— Dr A Naing, 234 Coldharbour Lane

Dentist: 3   Pharmacy: 3   Opticians: 1

Politicians   MP Terry Dicks (Conservative)
Councillors D Chand, C Rogers, S Saunders (Labour)

Public Transport   Buses: 195, H98, 90, 140, E6, U4, U6, N89
Hayes, Southall, Ealing, Hounslow, Northolt, Richmond, Heathrow Airport, Uxbridge

Leisure   Alfred Beck Leisure Centre, Town Hall Park

Places of Worship   Baptist Church, Hayes Christian Science, St Marys C of E, Hayes Town Chapel, Hayes Salvation Army and ignores earlier antecedents and more distant relations. It would therefore not be true to suggest that the Health Authority only started listening about concerns in Hayes early in 1996. Since 1994, the Health Authority and then FHSA have met bimonthly with GPs at convenient locations in the locality. Most Hayes GPs have attended at least once. The Health Authority also collaborated with the Local Authority, Citizens Advice Bureau and Community Health Council (CHC) in setting up and running a high street 'One Stop Shop' where people could obtain advice on a whole range of health matters at the same time as, say, consulting the CAB or paying their rent or Council Tax. The shop opened at the end of 1995.

However, the Health Authority's main focus had been acute service rationalisation in the North of the Borough. This included widespread informal and formal public consultation on the closure of the Accident and Emergency Department at Mount Vernon Hospital in favour of a Minor Injuries Unit and other service changes. That multi-agency consultation exercise was successful. The approach used there was adapted and adopted for use in Hayes.

At around the same time the Government launched its 'Primary Care Listening Exercise'. The Listening Exercise in Hillingdon was thorough and involved the following groups:

- Health Authority/FHSA Non Executives;
- GPs (Total Purchasing, Fundholding and non-Fundholding);
- Practice Managers;
- Practice Nurses;
- Trust Managers (Acute and Community);
- DHA/FHSA Managers;
- Clinic based Community Nurses and Therapist;
- Social Services;
- Community Health Council;
- Voluntary Organisations.

The exercise was extremely useful. We were aware of the views and frustrations of General Practitioners through the Locality Forums, and these were confirmed. However, what was extremely useful was to be able to sound out the views of other primary care staff, social services and the voluntary sector. It became evident that there were very different perceptions of the roles and responsibilities of the various professionals. By visiting many different professionals in a brief period, it was possible to feed in the views of others and facilitate closer contact. Particularly striking were the following:

- Most groups wanted to learn more about each others' skills and competencies and wanted to work more as a team. A Primary Care Team Building Exercise used extensively in Hayes ('*The Joint Ventures Initiative*') involved Social Services and the Voluntary Sector and drew universal acclaim. It was felt to be useful by other members of the Primary Care Team '... even if the GP was disengaged ...'
- Most staff felt their services under-resourced but that Social Services were worst off. It appeared that Social Services did not have a preventive role and that, for instance, a child would only be assigned a case worker after he had been abused. Health Visitors in particular felt that there was a gap between what they did and what Social Services did that needed filling. GPs had noted how many of their patients were front line Social Services staff finding it difficult to cope.
- Social Services reported that they felt that it was legitimate for Health Visitors to fill this void. They could not. They also expressed exasperation about the extent to which GPs could disrupt arrangements, especially because of Partnership disputes.
- The Voluntary Sector wanted to know why GPs ignored them and did not refer to the services they offered. Usually GPs were unaware that they existed. Voluntary organisations were unaware of stress levels in General Practice.

Also striking was the extent to which the 'blame culture' evaporated and to be replaced by sympathy and a willingness to collaborate when the problems of one group of primary care staff were explained to another group by a third party, in this instance the author.

The Hayes Listening Exercise built on this foundation by engaging far more with local people and their representatives. Painstaking community development work undertaken over the last 3 years by the Project Manager served as a very useful basis in accessing networks of interests throughout Hayes. Altogether about 100 statutory, voluntary, community and political organisations were invited to meet with or write to the Health Authority. The retiring local Conservative MP, with a majority of 55 was a controversial right-wing backbencher. All eight electoral wards have Labour Councillors. With evident political sensitivities at play, we have been scrupulous about our even-handedness and tried to focus on ethical issues rather than anything which might be portrayed as overtly political. This was particularly important as we were aware of the views of many local politicians that the Health Authority (and Trusts) lacked legitimacy because their non-Executive Members were unelected and accountable nationally rather than locally.

So far 45 meetings have been held and a number of written replies received. The meetings were held to suit those commenting. Traditionally, Health Authority organised meetings draw very thin audiences, but by asking to be put on the agenda of meetings already being held means that you can gauge a much wider range of opinion.

All the comments have been recorded. Because many of the comments go wider that health services, we are working with other agencies, especially the Local Authority, to identify opportunities to use the information gleaned. Recurring themes include:

- A wish to see GP, primary care and social services in Hayes strengthened and expanded to meet high levels of need and demand;
- Widespread concern about the effect of unemployment and other social factors on health, especially mental health;
- The need to target health promotion to those at greatest risk, with more accessible information about local services and diseases;
- More comprehensive and accessible mental health, counselling and support services especially for the socially isolated. Two particular estates were identified as areas of multiple deprivation and associated health problems (Willow Tree Lane and Cranford Park);
- Improved services for people from the minority ethnic communities, including refugees;
- Low morale in general practice, especially in relation to premises, recruitment, high demand for out-of-hours care/home visits and rising workload;
- Difficulty in accessing certain GPs, in some cases leading to inappropriate use of out-of-hours, A&E and even emergency ambulance services. However, several GPs believe their patients make inappropriate demands of their services;
- There is considerable local concern about air and noise pollution associated with the airport and the roads leading to it, perceived to be linked to high levels of asthma;
- That key sites in South Hayes would be useful for primary care developments;

- That NHS and local authority should consider supporting community development projects which involve and stem from local people.

Echoing the process which followed the national Primary Care Listening Exercise, the Hayes Health Plan now out for discussion is equivalent to *'Primary Care; The Future'*.[2] It says this is what we did, this is what we think we heard and these are the kind of opportunities for change we envisage. Before we firm up any plans are we on the right track?

PRIMARY CARE IN HAYES

There are presently 34 GPs in 18 practices with their main surgeries in Hayes. Ten practices are single handed, several from 'failed' partnerships. One third of the GPs are women. About 10 000 Hayes residents are registered with non-Hillingdon GPs, some 40% of whom registered with a practice which has a branch surgery in the middle of Hayes.

There were no GP fundholders in the first four waves, and only one in the fifth, but now just under half the population has a fundholding GP.

Demand for night visits is almost 50% higher than for the rest of Hillingdon.

GP recruitment has been increasingly difficult. There are currently two vacancies in Hayes. We therefore have to consider new and different ways of attracting high quality young doctors and developing new models of care. Possibilities include primary care centres providing a range of health and other services; more flexible career opportunities; salaried GPs and increased use of nurse practitioners. In this context the 1996 Primary Care White Papers came just at the right time for Hayes. It has been very encouraging to see one practice attract an additional partner with academic links anxious to provide 21st century medicine in a relatively deprived area from excellent new premises. Only a short time ago the partners appeared very cynical and demoralised. A Primary Care-Led NHS has breathed new life into their practice and such positive developments can be contagious.

The very positive response to the Joint Ventures Initiative aimed at creating wide primary care teams in an area where most of the GPs were single handed has been mentioned. However, it is much more difficult to create meaningful teams when so many of the premises have insufficient space and/or facilities for them to operate effectively.

Only three of the 19 surgeries in Hayes are of a good standard in terms of space, general condition and disability access; nine are adequate but could be improved. The remaining seven have been assessed as requiring improvements and in the case of four of them this would require a move to new premises. As mentioned elsewhere, uptake of certain primary care services is low in Hayes and this also tends to reflect poor premises.

It would be tempting to pretend that the impetus for strategic change in Hayes came from a consideration of wider service strategies. In the event it was pressure to improve individual premises that drew us to the conclusion that a strategic overview of health and healthcare was needed as a framework for future investment and collaboration with other agencies such as Social Services. A new health centre (The Warren) was built in North Hayes, using funds from the sale of the former District Headquarters building. The previous premises were essentially prefabs which leaked copiously whenever it rained. A similar health centre was proposed in South Hayes, using a special capital grant for deserving projects outside the London Initiative Zone. Proposals for health premises associated with the Single Regeneration Bid for the redevelopment of the Hayes and Harlington station site was an added impetus. At the same time the local Community Trust wished to rationalise its estate and four of its clinics are based in Hayes.

Community clinic services

Community clinics tend to flourish where the provision of maternal, family planning and child health services in general practice is less developed or where people prefer the clinics' services. They are often used to provide therapy services, dentistry and may serve as a base for health visitors, district nurses and school nurses.

A larger proportion of people in Hayes use community clinics, particularly for women's and children's services than elsewhere in the Borough. This reflects patient choice, the limited capacity of some local general practice and the high need for services. However, the clinics are not all necessarily located in the best places to meet the needs of the local populations. In addition social housing developments in the area will create new demands for health care which will need to be met. In discussion with the Local Authority there may be opportunities for joint provision of services, perhaps more locally, whilst releasing some land currently occupied by dilapidated clinics for these very social housing schemes. These issues and the particular circumstances of each clinic and the services provided from them form a key part of the discussion in the Hayes Health Plan.

Acute hospital services

The traditional boundaries between various health sectors are becoming increasingly blurred in a primary care-led NHS. So any strategic review of primary care needs to take account of acute services. The main acute provider for Hayes is the Hillingdon Hospital Trust which also provides Mental Health Services. Its Accident and Emergency Department, although just outside Hayes is probably *de facto* the biggest single primary care facility for the people of Hayes. Improved primary care in Hayes would therefore impact on the hospital. With increased fundholding there is increased pressure to provide outreach services in GP surgeries. To make the best use of available resources an outreach facility in central Hayes with good public transport links, such as the Hayes station site might make a range of services more locally accessible and by virtue of economies of scale could justify investment in, say, telemedicine.

A further issue at the interface between acute, primary and social care is the inappropriate use of hospital beds. Patients who could be cared for in primary settings if the services were available can often find themselves admitted via A&E, particularly elderly patients out-of-hours. A needs led assessment of such patients can take up to a week and thereafter there can be delays in arranging home care packages or admission to residential or nursing homes. The issue in relation to Hillingdon Hospital briefly, and largely inaccurately, made headline news in October 1996. The Health Authority is working very closely with Acute and Community Trusts, the Social Services Department and Primary Care to resolve the issue. Direct discussions between local GPs and Social Services have been held via the Locality Forums and there is a great deal of goodwill to re-engineer services to meet the total needs of local people, avoiding unnecessary and costly hospital admissions that prevent appropriate cases from getting in. There is much to be done.

The provision of mental health services on a locality basis is already well advanced with a new resource centre recently opened in Hayes. Again there are opportunities for jointly designing comprehensive services that bring together acute Trust, primary care and Social Services.

Local authority services

It is axiomatic that people have a range of needs as well as health needs. There are key interfaces with Social Services, Education, Housing, Leisure, the Police and so on. Designing services critically involves Local Authority planners with whom good relationships need to be forged if appropriate sites are to be found. A strategic overview needs to take account of all these services, not least because there may be opportunities to share facilities and provide more 'seamless' care. This process has already begun and has the potential to deliver very considerable benefits within available resources.

LESSONS LEARNED

There is widespread support for multi-agency working in primary care but it can be extremely time consuming and progress is disappointingly slow. Change of key personnel and organisational structures can further slow the process. But the approach taken to look at the whole picture, share information and feedback and integrate both consultation and community development activities makes sense to all concerned. The forging of an ethical consensus and the active involvement of key stakeholders in a Project Steering Group has been warmly welcomed and is likely to endure. The Primary Care White Papers once enacted will provide opportunities to improve the quality and range of primary care for this population. There are clearly problems which need to be addressed at the interface between primary and social care. But these are not insuperable. Good work has been done and that should provide a sound foundation, regardless of further management changes or the political complexion of central or local Government. Because the approach relies on continuing commitment from all parties it must lead to concrete improvements or it will lead to disaffection. The advantage it does have is to generate a debate about health and related issues which can raise public awareness in advance of decisions. As such it improves the chances of broad-based support for the changes which emerge from the process.

REFERENCES

1. Secretary of State for Health Primary Care: The Future. Choice and Opportunity (October 1996) and Delivering the Future (December 1996). HMSO, London
2. Secretary of State for Health (June 1996), Primary Care: The Future. NHSE, London

5. The Bournemouth Experience: Care in the community for elderly people

Diana Churchill and Geoff Colvin

No book of this kind would be complete without a contribution from Dorset, the bravest innovator in contemporary health and social care. But not the most foolhardy: as this chapter shows, the message is not collaboration at all costs. In tackling the major demographic challenge together and seeking to combine frontline services for elderly people in primary care settings the health and local authorities have gained some hard-headed lessons about the VFM dividend — or lack of. The project management costs are high; the nursing skills mix is excessive, and care management would seem to be an efficient option in general practice only if applied across all client groups. Simply improving local inter-professional goodwill and understanding is not good enough.

SEASIDE SOCIETY

Bournemouth has an image of being a genteel seaside town full of well-to-do old ladies taking afternoon tea, enjoying the warm, rather un-English climate and listening to Radio 4. While there is undoubtedly a high proportion of elderly people living in Bournemouth, they are certainly not all well-to-do and there are many other groups characterising the town; which is today a lively, somewhat cosmopolitan conurbation with a University, many foreign language schools and a well developed tourist industry.

While essentially an affluent area, Bournemouth has its fair share of social problems, including those associated with isolated council housing estates, areas of multi-occupancy housing and elderly owner occupiers whose wealth is tied up in their homes and who have great difficulty making ends meet on their current incomes. Certain wards in Bournemouth score high on the Jarman[1] index and there are areas notorious for drug misuse and petty crime.

From 1 April 1997 Bournemouth, which lost both its county borough status and historical association with the county of Hampshire in 1974, once again becomes responsible, as a new unitary authority, for the services currently provided by Dorset County Council such as Social Services and Education. What this means for the citizens of Bournemouth has yet to be revealed but the opportunity to regain the town as an independent entity has been eagerly embraced by the local politicians, and enthusiasm and optimism abound.

THE DORSET DIMENSION

Bournemouth, as a part of Dorset County Council Social Services Department, has for some years, enjoyed a close and productive relationship with the Dorset Health Authority. The Authority has a national reputation for encouraging innovative developments in primary care. In 1993 it was agreed by the two agencies that a series of projects should be set up to test different ways of purchasing health and social care in primary care settings. Six practices in Dorset were chosen to participate and a slightly different model was piloted in each one. The idea was that either health service staff in general practices would be enabled to purchase social care for their patients, or that social services staff would be enabled to purchase health care for their clients. The direct costs of the projects were funded by Dorset Health Authority.

This objective proved to be rather ambitious. It was straightforward enough to enable health service staff to purchase social care as all this required was to set up systems to allow them to effectively operate as care managers and access the appropriate social care budget. It was less straightforward to enable social care staff to access health budgets. Health care staff in general practice are providers rather than purchasers and there was therefore, no readily accessible budget which could be accessed to purchase health care, even if it was accepted that social services staff were able to make decisions about what health care needed to be purchased, which was debatable. It was therefore decided to compromise on the original objective and to think in terms of social services staff becoming members of primary health care teams which would allow them immediate and appropriate access to health care for their clients if this was felt to be needed.

THE PROJECTS

The six projects took place in various locations throughout Dorset. Two practices were not typical in that they already employed social workers using funding allocated to them by Dorset Health Authority as part of its primary care development programme. The key element of these projects was that these social workers were enabled to access the social services community care budgets which had not been the case before. Of the remaining four projects, two involved a social services care manager being based in a practice and two involved health service staff, for example the district nurse, being enabled to access the local community care budgets.

It proved impossible to start all six projects at the same time because of the difficulty of recruiting enough interested practices and the sheer logistics of having enough time to devote to setting up each project, which, as is often the case with schemes of this kind, took longer than anticipated. While practice staff were invariably interested and enthusiastic the introduction of the projects meant changes in ways of working which needed explaining and working through. The projects also meant increased work for the local social services team managers, who, while they gained the advantage of additional care managers in their teams, also gained the workload implications of having to supervise and support what were, in effect, additional members of staff. In some projects, although not in the Bournemouth schemes, computers were installed in the practices and in all cases where health service staff took on the care management role, there was a need for intensive training in using the social services computer system. This was very time consuming.

The effect of this was that the first project, which was the North Bournemouth project, began in May 1994 and finished in May 1995, while the last project to begin, a project in Poole based around a district nurse undertaking the role of care manager, started in May 1996 and finished in March 1997.

EVALUATION ISSUES

The issue of the timescale has had an unhelpful impact on the evaluation of the project. At the outset it was recognised that any evaluation would not meet the criteria of a rigorous research exercise as there were no controls in place and no funding available to employ outside evaluators. However, it was considered to be very important that some kind of evaluation took place and an evaluation protocol was drawn up which identified key benchmarks against which the projects would be judged by a small team of both health and social services staff involved in the projects. The benchmarks were issues such as the quality of the service offered, including the content of care plans, costs of the services provided, the workload of the project workers and the benefits to the primary health care team. All of these indicators were to be compared with the outcome of similar work undertaken by social services care managers based in the local office. The project workers have all kept detailed records and statistical information on the work they have undertaken in order to allow comparisons to be made. In very basic terms, the benchmarks were designed to show whether or not the projects delivered benefit both to the patients and carers and to the agencies involved and whether there was any one model which seemed to be more beneficial than the others.

The elongated timescale of the projects has meant that comparisons between each project became more and more questionable because time in the community care field does not stand still and there have been many developments in social services and in the health service over the last few years, some of which have been influenced by the lessons learnt from the early projects and some of which would have happened anyway. In addition, in some cases there has been a need to make a judgement as to whether the model established in a particular practice, which has proved popular and is perceived to be working well, should be allowed to continue after the end of the project rather than dismantle the arrangements and wait for an evaluation to pronounce on whether or not it had been successful. Despite these problems, the project team has endeavoured to evaluate each project according to the original protocol and there will be a final report later in 1997 drawing conclusions from all of the schemes after the last one has been completed.

NORTH BOURNEMOUTH

One of each of the two types of project was based in Bournemouth. The North Bournemouth locality project involved a senior nurse undertaking care management for three practices in the area while the Beaufort Road surgery practice involved a half-time social services care manager being based in the practice as a member of the primary health care team. In the North Bournemouth project there was an issue about boundaries since two of the practices covered parts of Poole as well as Bournemouth where the responsibility for the social services budgets were with different social services teams. It was therefore decided to restrict the patients eligible for the project to those who were under the auspices of the North Bournemouth social services team. This meant that in one of the practices 53% of the patients were included in the project and in the second practice 66%.

The two projects were based in very different areas with different problems. The practice profiles of the three practices in North Bournemouth indicate a predominantly young population while the Beaufort Road practice, which is in Southbourne, has a profile of mainly elderly people. The North Bournemouth area is mixed in terms of socio-economic profile but there is a relatively high level of unemployment and a significant proportion of young families with low incomes. There are very few residential or nursing homes in the vicinity of the three North Bournemouth practices whereas Southbourne has the highest concentration in Bournemouth.

A decision had been taken at the start of these two projects to restrict the care management function to the elderly services budget, primarily for practical reasons. The majority of care management at that time was concerned with elderly people and it was felt that project control and monitoring would be easier if the relationship of the practice care manager was with one team manager and one budget. In both projects however, there was an expectation that the practice-based project worker would act as a liaison worker for the rest of social services and that all referrals to social services would be channelled through her. This proved to be a very successful and valued element of both projects.

In the event, the focus on the elderly care budget may not have been the most fruitful approach in the case of the North Bournemouth project since the number of elderly people requiring care management is relatively low. During the first year of the project, the nurse care manager dealt with 249 referrals compared with 162 referrals at the Southbourne practice. However, the number of full assessments carried out in the North Bournemouth project was 13 whereas the number in the Southbourne project was 50. This reflects a high proportion of referrals in the North Bournemouth practice that were not for elderly care services. It may have been more beneficial in hindsight to have designed the North Bournemouth project around the need for social work interventions with families, children and vulnerable adults, rather than exclusively on older people.

A key difference between the projects was that the care manager in North Bournemouth was a senior nurse and the care manager in the Southbourne project was a social services care manager. The senior nurse is actually employed by one of the three practices involved in the scheme as a nurse team leader responsible for managing the work of the practice-based community nurses and the practice nurses. This takes up about 12 hours of her time each week and for the rest of the time she is the care manager for the three practices in the project, relating to a team manager in the North Bournemouth Social Services Local Office.

The North Bournemouth pilot has finished as a project but the practices have negotiated to retain the services of the project worker and she is continuing to undertake her role on the basis of part nurse team leader and part care manager. The fact that the practices involved were keen to retain the service is evidence that the project was successful and valued. However, the evaluation of the project which was undertaken internally by staff from Dorset Social Services Department and Dorset Health Authority, while recognising the benefits which the arrangement brought to the practices involved, also concluded that the model had some drawbacks, the primary one being that it is relatively expensive. The evaluation concluded that the fact that the care manager was a nurse did not substantially alter the type or cost of the service provided to the patients who were being care managed and that there was, therefore, no compelling reason why the role could not be just as adequately performed by a care manager who would cost less than a senior nurse. This conclusion was in no way a reflection on the competence of the particular individual involved, whose contribution and expertise are highly valued, but a realistic assessment of the hard economics of the case.

SOUTHBOURNE

This conclusion has been borne out by the preliminary evaluation of the Southbourne project which finished at the end of 1996. The contribution of the care manager has been enormous with the general practitioners saying that her presence has been one of the most beneficial things ever to happen in the practice. This view is clearly affected by the fact that the practice has such a high proportion of elderly patients. This part of Bournemouth has a high concentration of residential and nursing homes and the care manager's input into assessments and admissions to these has been invaluable to the practice. In addition many of the elderly patients want to remain at home for as long as possible and the care manager has set up appropriate packages of care, often with high levels of support. While social services care managers are successfully undertaking these roles in other localities for other Dorset residents, the Southbourne practice staff would argue that the process is easier and more efficient and that both the patients and carers receive an enhanced and more personal service when the care manager is one of the primary health care team. The project has meant a much closer level of cooperation between the general practitioners and social services as well as closer working between the other members of the primary health care team which has led to a far greater understanding of both the constraints and the opportunities within which each set of professionals is working. The practice is unequivocal that this has led to an enhanced service to their patients, particularly because one of the impacts has been a lowering of the referral threshold to social services enabling a preventive approach to be taken which, in turn, reduces the amount of crisis intervention work needed.

Although not a nurse, the care manager has on one or two occasions identified unmet health care needs which she has enabled her practice colleagues to deal with. She has also been a valuable resource to the practice in terms of being able to give instant expert advice and information on social services legislation and practice.

An interesting aspect of the evaluation has been the similarity in the costs of the care packages set up by both the health and social services professionals. Unfortunately, it has not been possible to undertake any work on the outcomes of the various interventions made and whether there is any difference in outcomes depending on the background of the assessor. Nor has it been possible to ascertain the views of patients and carers. At the beginning of the evaluation there was a good deal of discussion as to whether it was possible to obtain the views of patients and carers but it was concluded that it was difficult to ask people whether they preferred a particular model of service to another when they would have had no experience of the other model. It was concluded, rightly or wrongly, that the only kind of question it would have been possible to ask would be along the lines of whether the patient/carer had felt satisfied with the service or not and it was considered that the added value to the purpose of the evaluation from this information did not justify the time or resource that it would have taken to obtain it.

Key benefits

One of the undoubted benefits of both projects has been the increased understanding and awareness of the role of social services by the members of the primary health care teams and particularly by general practitioners. General practitioners and social services traditionally do not mix very well and there tends to be a certain amount of distrust and suspicion on both sides. The need to work closely together in getting these projects off the ground and to solve mutual problems has been of enormous benefit. This has been true despite changes of key personnel on the social services side because of reorganisation or promotion.

An important factor in maintaining enthusiasm and momentum for the projects has been the involvement of the Project Officer-Health and Community Care, who works for Dorset Social Services. This is a jointly funded post and the individual concerned was a district nurse before joining social services. This gives her credibility with the health service staff and her input has been extremely valuable, particularly with regard to evaluation of the projects.

While both Bournemouth projects have been enormously valuable learning experiences, there is no doubt that the practice based care manager seems to offer the most transferable and cost-effective model to take forward in the future, particularly in areas where there is a large population of elderly people. The two projects were not directly comparable because of the differences in population and there is certainly scope for developing different types of practice based models of social services provision in more mixed population areas. It has yet to be seen how the new unitary local authority, along with Dorset Health Authority and local general practitioners, will pick up the challenge of building a practice based approach to the purchasing and provision of both health and social care for the residents of Bournemouth.

REFERENCE

1. Jarman B 1983 Identification of Underprivileged Areas. British Medical Journal 286: pp 1705–1709

6. The Trowbridge Experience: Care in the community for elderly people

Stephen Henry and Lynn Gaskin

This chapter maintains the focus of the previous one on elderly care, but takes it much further. Driven by a leadership conviction, particularly in the Social Services Department, that fully integrated services are the way forward and supported by a particularly democratic style of general practice, Chapter 6 is genuinely 'leading edge'. The range of service collaboration and innovation is extremely impressive; the investment in staffing to make the necessary 'links' is unique and the role of the GP, unexpectedly, for many, generous and positive. But this is no ordinary GP: Stephen Henry is one of Fundholding's foremost founding fathers; the market towns of Wiltshire are perhaps the most natural pilot sites for service development in the country and, for many Directors of Social Services, Trowbridge would still be an anathema. There is a great deal of transferable learning in the pages that follow but the need for more universal policy, management and organisational frameworks remains.

HISTORY IN THE MAKING

There has been a certain inevitability in the continuing drive to incorporate a main stream social care element into the daily business of General Practice in Wiltshire. Prior to 1990 district (community) nurses and health visitors had been attached to practices in Wiltshire both geographically and specifically in turn. Personal alliances and allegiances built up as relationships developed between GPs and these attached staff, but clear cut demarcation lines of who could do what and who could not remained. Although there were identified adult and child team social workers officially related to individual practices, access to social services was usually through the duty officer. Yet another social worker was based at the community hospital, serving all the practices which had admitting rights. The liaison was poor. Few GPs knew who was who or who was responsible for what. Staff were constantly changing. Cultural and organisational barriers were well entrenched. Service — something actually happening — seemed to take forever and requests for help appeared to disappear in a morass of committee indecision. Meanwhile in the GP surgeries, consultations began to become increasingly social in context as opposed to clinical, to such an extent that in 1982 the Lovemead Practice in Trowbridge engaged a retired senior mental welfare officer on a part-time basis to deal at least with the crisis elements as they occurred, relieving the GPs and the primary health care team (PHCT) of involvement in the difficult social, financial and housing problems with which they were neither trained nor inclined to cope. When he finally retired, an attempt was made to replace him with a secondment directly from social services but the overall cost together with difficulties of arranging shared duties with other practices proved insurmountable.

LINKING LOVEMEAD, TROWBRIDGE AND WILTSHIRE

The Lovemead Group Practice is one of four practices in Trowbridge, (population 37 000), all now fundholding. It looks after approximately one third of the local population. Wiltshire's only first wave fundholders (1991), the practice is now part of a Total Purchasing Pilot (1995) which includes one other Trowbridge practice, the Adcroft Surgery. Together they form the majority purchasers for the town. Out of a practice list size of 14 200, the practice has 2150 patients who are over 65. Of these 1155 are between 65 and 75 and 995 over 75 years old.

Following the central policy initiatives on Community Care in the early 1990s the local impetus was revived. Wiltshire Family Health Services Authority, (FHSA) had developed an early model of practice-based assessment and 'commissioning' before its merger with the Bath District Health Authority into the Bath and Wiltshire Health Commission (now reduced to the Wiltshire Health Authority). This resulted in the Linkworker scheme. Drawn from a variety of professional backgrounds (nurses, health visitors or social workers etc.) and jointly funded by the FHSA and Social Services Department, linkworkers are tasked with the development of care management in the primary care setting. The Director of Wiltshire

Social Services backed this approach of encouraging adult social care teams to work more closely with local GP practices and other primary care colleagues (for reasons well described by Yvonne Wilkin and Ralph Heywood in Chapter 11) aided by pressure from well organised local users and carers networks.

Lovemead successfuly bid for a linkworker, engaging a nurse already employed by the practice to carry out the over-75 assessments. A health visitor by background, she was resourced for additional hours as a linkworker to take on care management for the practice's adult patients for 75% of her additional time, with 25% spent in a 'linking' role. She received supervision from the social services adult care team manager, and became a member of both the PHCT and the social services adult care team. Monitoring of the linkworker placement was overseen by a practice steering group with the assistance of a county development worker. Support and care management training for linkworkers was provided at county level with joint funding. Initially, the arrival of the linkworker was greeted with sceptisism by the GPs. The notion of social services and health working side by side was somewhat alien and these two cultures needed to be reconciled. Meetings held with staff and GPs in the practice, explaining the roles and responsibilities of the linkworker and the aims and objectives laid out, did little in the early days to convince the PHCT. It was by demonstration and practical application of the assessments, and follow through of the care management role, that her impact began to be felt. Development of 'Link Lunches' organised and chaired by the linkworker helped to de-mystify her role. These lunches, held every 2 months, brought together groups of people from a variety of agencies engaged in community care in its widest sense. They included users and carers, members of the statutory organisations, representatives of private care providers and voluntary services. Held in the surgery, on an informal basis, the GPs became familiar with their style and began appreciating their worth. The presence of the linkworker and her assistant gradually increased the awareness in the practice of the implications of community care and how, by having a practice-based social link team, the continuity of care for the older population could be enhanced.

Formal evaluation of the project by Bath University[1] agreed that a nurse, supervised by social services, can operate effectively in a care management role. However, while providing a good bridge, the authors expressed doubt that the project had actually narrowed the gap between primary health and social care. For example, they said that while all GPs felt they knew more about social provision generally than they had before, they welcomed linkworking not so much because of that but because it allowed them to hand work across to social services more smoothly and with greater confidence that something would happen as a result. Linkworking seems to have improved coordination, but on its own may not be capable of promoting the integration of health and social care, i.e. seamless care.

PRIMARY CARE-LED PURCHASING — A NEW ERA

The impact on the practice of becoming first wave fundholders in 1991 was considerable. The contracted community nurses and health visitors moved into the surgery. After an initial conflict over 'ownership', the practice settled into a period of adjustment and cooperation between professionals, used to working together, but at arm's length from each other. The provider Community Trust reshaped their management structure accordingly. A layer of middle management was removed, enabling a release of funds for additional nursing hours. This was the beginning of a new era. The GPs, used to a relatively introspective existence, now found themselves co-existing with community nurses, health visitors, physiotherapists, chiropodists, counsellors, masseurs, osteopaths and audiology technicians. New services developed from a carefully considered strategic plan. The health visitors pioneered a children's triage clinic to run each day in conjunction with the GPs and the district nurses set up continence and leg ulcer clinics alongside the existing practice nurse-run clinics. The counsellor took referrals to help deal with the worried well and developed an anxiety management group, while the physiotherapist embarked upon a back pain clinic. By the time the suggestion was put forward to include social service staff in the practice, (see below) the PHCT was suffering from a degree of innovation fatigue! The idea of an integrated health and social team was viewed somewhat sceptically. However, by reasoned argument, presentations by the health and social care team and gentle persuasion, the practice agreed to the pilot scheme going ahead.

The progression to Total Purchasing in 1995 added two new dimensions. First, the practice was able to purchase its own beds. Notably, the cost of low intensity beds is the same as high intensity ones, even in the community hospital, so the opportunity was taken to purchase a bed in a nearby nursing home for the sole use of the practice at a fraction of the cost. This matched another bed purchased by the Health Authority for general GP respite care and a third purchased by social services for social respite. Second, came the appointment of a Primary Care Liaison Manager (PCLM). This is an experienced nurse practitioner who visits all the practice patients in hospital on a daily basis, ensuring that planned treatment happens on time, encouraging and facilitating the discharge process from admission, liaising with the health and social team as well as involving the patients, their relatives and carers in a smooth passage through hospital and back into the community. There are minimal delays and minimal bed blocking. The patients are very appreciative of the fact that their doctor has sent someone along to see them. 'Even though I haven't seen a doctor' said one elderly lady in the community hospital, 'at least he knows what's happening to me'. Patients being discharged from acute hospitals by the PCLM may return to the Practice's nursing home bed for postoperative rehabilitation etc. or continuing 'social' care rather than the community hospital. In this fashion, the boundaries of 'care' and payment for social/health care are becoming blurred. The tightening of admission protocols in this way has improved the service to patients as well as actually realising a cost saving of more than the PCLM's salary.

ENTER THE KINGS FUND AND INNOVATION

In 1993 the Kings Fund invited bids for participants in a nationwide project to help health and social care agencies purchase and provide services to meet the needs of older people and their carers.

Lovemead Group Practice and the Social Services Adult Care Team (West) began their joint project with an emphasis on practice based joint commissioning; links between strategic and operational levels in both the health authority and the social services; and the involvement of older people.

A multi-disciplinary steering group was set up to manage the project and create the network. The members included an elderly patient and a carer from the practice, representatives of the Users and Carers Networks, health and social services personnel, together with a GP from the practice and the Social Services Department's adult care team manager. Strategic staff from the Health Authority and SSD attended the meetings on a regular basis.

Meetings and workshops were held in the local area to see how older people could be involved in the project and to begin to indicate the priorities for service development. A local needs assessment was carried out. This research identified three main areas of unmet need:

- Affordable domestic help
- Flexible transport
- Information

At the same time a development worker was appointed to consult further with users and carers, identify gaps in services and recommend new services, or the adjustment of existing ones.

The involvement of older people and their carers took place through informal discussions at luncheon clubs, day centres, residents' associations and at the practice patients' forum etc. Reference was made to other local needs assessment exercises including 'Healthier Trowbridge', a 3-year health and safety initiative, and the 1994 Community Health Council/Council of Voluntary Services 'Spotlight on health and care services for older people'. Links were also made to the Trowbridge Local Health Plan and information was collated from the Practice's over-75 assessments. Thanks to the foresight of the Health Authority, the 5 years of information from these compulsory health checks included written records of social and functional status as well as medical, from the state of teeth, hearing and incontinence, to mobility and social contacts, self-awareness and benefit uptake; a genuine record of handicap and disability.

To build up the specification, a 'mapping and gapping' exercise of services available was carried out. Gaps were identified and the possibilities for reshaping or developing new services were explored. Links to service priorities at a strategic level were made and service possibilities discussed with both the steering group and local providers. The network was expanded to include the District Council, voluntary groups and the coterminous Community Trusts. Funding opportunities were explored and in one development option, application made for Joint Finance.

New services

Examples of developments now being pursued are outlined below.

'Handihelp West Wilts'

This is an alliance formed by the District Council, the Health Authority, the Social Services Department, the voluntary organisations and some practices, with users and carers, (through joint finance and Healthy Alliances) to provide practical help for the elderly and disabled. It includes house maintenance and repairs where residents cannot manage them and suitable alterations for security and accident prevention.

Gardening service

A local voluntary group has been contracted to provide a service for a pilot period.

Affordable Domestic Assistance (ADA)

A central register (with Age Concern) of self-employed individuals willing to carry out low cost domestic help for the elderly and their carers is being explored.

Community care and health information leaflet

Following discussions with practice patients and a joint agency group, this signposting leaflet has been developed for all 65–75-year-old patients with information on everything from leisure and counselling services through self-care to voluntary and statutory organisations.

Other developments

With finance from the Kings Fund, the Practice's Service Quality Initiative project worker and the linkworker have organised carer awareness training and carer identification, and arranged for the Practice newsletter to include 'Senior Snippets' of community information. The information sources within the Practice have been expanded to include DSS benefits information, a voluntary organisations and self-help groups database and a link to the Social Service Department's database. The national Help for Health information service is also available, via computer, in the surgery waiting room.

WORKING TOGETHER: THE THREE DIMENSIONS

1. The Health and Social Care Team

This is a joint agency team with a practice aligned social worker, serving the practice population of older people, younger physically disabled adults and their respective carers. The core team (Box 6.1) is led by the Assistant Adult Care Team Manager and is managed by a management steering group (Box 6.2). They commissioned an outside consultancy firm to facilitate team building and to support and guide the team to achieve its aims and objectives through implementation of care management mechanisms and processes. Together the team and consultant are looking for improved methods of working across agency boundaries and to slowly move from cooperation towards genuine integration.

Box 6.1

```
              CORE
      HEALTH AND SOCIAL TEAM
    Assistant Adult Care Team Manager
           (Coordinator role)
              Social Worker
             District Nurses
               Linkworker
           Assistant Linkworker
          Occupational Therapist
              Assistant O.T.
```

```
            NON CORE MEMBERS
           General Practitioners
       Primary Care Liaison Manager
              Physiotherapist
        Community Psychiatric Nurse
```

Box 6.2

```
         HEALTH AND SOCIAL CARE
             MANAGEMENT TEAM
          Practice General Manager
    Social Services Adult Care Team Manager
         Community Trust Nurse Manager
            General Practitioner
             Development Worker
                    User
              User Support Worker
                    Carer
              Carer Support Worker
```

2. The programme

The Team are now based together in one room, in the GP surgery. Users and carers have drawn up a list of desired outcomes which they would wish to see from the integrated team. Following workshops facilitated by the independent consultancy firm, the health and social care team have used these to set their task objectives.

Stage one tasks

'Tasked inter-agency groups' are to tackle immediate issues:

- Siting the staff together;
- Discrete administrative support;
- Transfer and storage of social services and nursing records;
- Confidentiality;
- Joint records in the home;
- Protocols for allocation of referrals to an appropriate worker;
- Maintaining social services duty cover;
- Roles of team co-ordinator, management steering group and line managers;
- Support to social services staff;
- Equity implications for remaining town population.

Stage two tasks

These will address issues such as:

- Additional teambuilding;
- Access to each other's training;
- Joint assessment forms;
- Joint resource shortfall monitoring; links with other agencies and teams, i.e. housing, mental health, community hospitals and the voluntary sector.

3. Contracting and commissioning

Historical practice level spending has been identified by both the Practices and the Social Services Department. The budget holders are the SSD's Adult Care Manager and the total fundholding practice. To reshape and develop services, the differing contracting mechanisms have had to be taken into consideration. At different stages legal and financial advice has been sought from contracting and commissioning experts within the different agencies and the Practice. Section 28A of the NHS Act 1977 was used to make application for Joint Finance linked to the priorities and objectives set out in a Community Care Plan. In addition, aligned budgets between the practice and the adult care team are being considered. There is, of course, difficulty in melding health and social services budgets, free for health but means tested for social services. If the Practice wishes to purchase on its own account, there is the difficulty of disaggregating a percentage of already active Health Authority contracts to release cash for new primary care initiatives to be shared with social services. This can only be done by a reduction in activity on funds already committed to provide current work and then it may be only at marginal rates. The SSD practice budget is almost entirely committed to residential and nursing home care as is the practice budget to hospital and community health care.

In fact the Practice General Manager has managed to separate some 5% of the historical spend on major providers to support the PCLM and other costs of total purchasing as well as a small cash float for cross boundary use by the health and social team. Likewise, the Adult Care Team Manager has secured a small 'initiative' allowance from his locality budget for similar use. The Team has in reality become the purchaser of community care for the practice as well as social services, with direct access to the 'joint' budget and will review the opportunities for disinvestment and reinvestment as new needs arise, for there is certainly no new money about.

Evidence so far suggests much quicker response times and less duplication for workers, users and carers. Case studies reflect prevention of hospital admission due to earlier referral to the occupational therapist, and social care issues being identified at an earlier stage.

Evaluation is being carried out, again in conjunction with Bath University.

Spreading our wings

From 1996 Department of Health funding has been awarded for 2 years under the 'Building Partnerships for Success' community care development programme to expand the work to include the other total purchasing practice and the two remaining fundholding practices in the town.

This funding will allow the development worker to continue in post and build upon the joint commissioning work already undertaken. The aims are to further involve older people and to show how they can have a real influence on service development and at the same time to explore the impact on service provision of the differing purchasing powers of the fundholding/total purchasing practices together with devolved social services budgets within the locality. Workshops have so far identified priorities for further discussion including closer links being made to local health planning groups and closer involvement with providers.

Work has started on a guide to a detailed health and social care *Locality* purchasing plan for older peoples services, with a breakdown of a 'snapshot' community care spend for each Practice's population. Alignment of budgets is still under discussion. Individual practices have indicated specific initiatives for collaborative work with social services focusing on their older population. These include:

- Joint planning with social services;
- Practice-based social services staff;
- Hospital admission and discharge services and protocols;
- Integration of the teams;
- Social care and the over-75 assessment;
- Health and social care information for the 65–75 age group;
- Pro-active information and services to carers;
- Giving pro-active benefits information.

Older people's groups are being set up for feedback on locality based needs assessments. These groups are being recognised as an integral part of the health and social services locality planning structures. The first meeting was attended by over 130 older people. General Practices and social services adult care will be kept informed of the results of the needs assessment for planning and service provision purposes.

FUTURE RIDDLES

Richard Poxton,[2] the project manager of the national Kings Fund project, has written:
Of the five development sites, Wiltshire is by far the most committed to a locally based approach to needs assessment and determining what responses should be made.

He cites leadership at both local and strategic levels as a principal reason.

It is difficult to escape the contrast of styles. With a line management structure, Wiltshire Social Services appear to have been driven towards integration by their Director, Dr Ray Jones, from the top and at times faster than middle management or team members wished to go. On the other hand, General Practices are organisationally democratic, at least at partner level. The health and social team members seem to have hijacked what might have been considered the doctor's agenda from relatively 'disengaged' GPs. This may be partly due to the closed shop nature of General Practice, partly the perverse incentive of current general medical services funding, whereby more staff equals less take-home pay for GPs.

When the full implications of joint purchasing and budgetary management impinge on the 'board of partners', it is interesting to speculate what degree of re-engagement may be expected, with what effect on the team itself and to what extent the development of the three additional practice team mimics the progress of the original. Whether they can ever work cohesively together as a genuine integrated locality service for the whole town remains the ultimate enigma.

REFERENCES

1. Challis L, Pearson J 1994 The Lovemead Linkworker Project. School of Social Sciences, University of Bath
2. Poxton R 1996 Joint approaches for a better old age. Kings Fund, London

7. The County Durham Experience: From primary health services to primary care teams

Pauline Murray

In the context of the 1997 Primary Care legislation which prefaces the development of new types of primary care organisation in the UK, the Durham experience is particularly pertinent. Pauline Murray illustrates how, within the same county, different environmental factors can appropriately lead to different integrated primary care team arrangements, focused on both a particular local area or an individual client group; for either operational or planning purposes in terms of service delivery. For the first time in this book the major impact of technological advances in driving health and local authorities to pursue together the more efficient use of resources in community settings is considered.

THE ROAD TO DEVOLUTION

Over recent years the County Durham Social Services Department has developed and established a range of models within localities to support and strengthen links with Primary Care Teams. The paper begins by considering the background of past and current issues in order to establish the context of these models.

Since 1990, decision making budgetary control and management have been devolved to the operational level. A restructuring in 1993 in response to Community Care legislative requirements endorsed and reinforced this pattern of decentralisation. The commissioning branch of the department has adopted a specialist team approach in which care managers and social workers practise within localities. These geographically defined areas are broadly coterminous with local District Councils and the purchasing

Localities established by the County Durham Health Authority. There is, therefore, a ready made vehicle for locally based joint planning and joint commissioning. Each specialist team is led by a Team Manager who controls the purchase of care budget for the specialism in that locality. In addition to purchasing individual care packages, Team Managers are able to promote service developments in response to service mapping and unmet need. Accordingly, there exists across the County a wide range of service agreements which are responsive to local circumstances and demographic patterns. Gate keeping for residential and nursing home care and high level domiciliary care packages are through local resource allocation panels. The department is not prescriptive in its composition and membership is a matter for local determination.

The continuing care debate has inevitably impacted upon Health and Social Services creating the potential for disputes over financial responsibility for care. The two agencies continue to work together at senior management level to achieve the goal of jointly agreed criteria. Locally the panels provide a forum for decision making and debate wherever possible reflecting the shared view that problem solving and resolution should be a matter for operational staff. The key to responsive care planning which informs financial responsibility is comprehensive, multi-disciplinary assessment in which Primary Care Team members are committed partners.

Following the implementation of the 1990 NHS and Community Care Act, Health and Social Services have faced fundamental structural and organisational changes. Ostensibly both Health and Social Services Authorities operate a purchaser/provider split. While this is undoubtedly so, there are significant differences between the two. As purchasers of health care for populations Health Authorities negotiate major block contracts with the NHS Trusts. Their market is largely internal. By contrast, Social Services Care Management processes are within a mixed market of independent, voluntary sector and in house provision and focus upon the needs of the individual where care packages are spot purchased. Opportunities for both agencies to consolidate operational and planning arrangements have been limited in a climate of frequent change and financial restriction. A range of issues has emerged and must now be addressed. Local Authorities continue to be confronted by ongoing financial constraints exacerbated by a high level of demand for Community

Care support and increasing public expectations. Demographic trends show an increasingly elderly population. The Department's stated priorities must therefore give precedence to those with the highest levels of need. Some authorities like Durham have also been faced with boundary changes through local government review.

THE PRIMARY IMPERATIVE

Technological advances in health care move patients inexorably from secondary to primary care services. GPs are becoming increasingly alarmed by the additional demands placed upon them. Targets aimed at reducing length of patient stay reinforce the trend of shorter in-patient care, earlier discharge and reliance on day treatment and surgery. Tension is inevitable as Health Authorities struggle to manage the competing demands of secondary and primary care. The changing patterns in the traditional balance of care have the potential to increase mistrust. There are crucial issues which must be faced openly and honestly if real joint working and planning are to happen. In many ways Primary Care Teams occupy the central ground — at best key influencers and shapers — at worst caught in the cross fire.

There is a lack of consensus about even the term Primary Care Team with no universally agreed definition of membership. In many instances the different professionals who make up the team do not share accommodation or co-location. Management arrangements for individual team members are significantly different. GPs are seen to enjoy comparative autonomy; community nurses are generally employees of NHS Trusts; specialist advisors may be hospital based and care managers work for the Local Authority. The purchasing potential of Fundholding Practices may reshape even this disjointed pattern. Staff experience differing organisational and cultural frameworks and yet must work together if they are to achieve shared goals. Primary care encompasses purchaser and provider functions. It occupies a pivotal role between community and secondary care and is instrumental in directing people to, and receiving them from, other care settings.

It is against this background that a number of models have developed in County Durham. All seek to promote a multi-agency response to local and individual need. It is over prescriptive to suggest that there is one 'right' model for effective primary care working. Each must be responsive to local circumstances, making best use of available resources. However, broad aims must be to avoid inappropriate institutional solutions to care needs, to avoid duplication of effort, to be flexible and responsive and make effective use of the available skill mix within the team. Inter-agency Primary Care Teams offer the potential for effective gate keeping, prioritisation and resource allocation. The County Durham models share the objectives of establishing multi-disciplinary processes, responsive case management and the development of robust communication channels.

THE EASINGTON MODEL

The one stop shop

Joint planning arrangements in Easington locality are through a Joint Commissioning Board (JCB) which includes membership from the Social Services Department, the Health Authority, the District Council and a local GP. The JCB established Local Advisory Groups consisting of agency staff, members of voluntary organisations and local people, some of whom were service users or their carers. In 1994, facilitated by the Kings Fund Centre, the JCB arranged a search conference bringing together almost 100 professionals and lay people from across a broad spectrum. The Conference, held over 2 days, was designed to consider the current situation, reflect on how the future would look if nothing changed, create a vision for a different future and identify the first steps in an action plan for change. When considering the current position the following key themes emerged:

- There was a lack of information for local people;
- There was poor inter-agency communication leading to duplication and gaps;
- There was poor access to care agents. In a locality with several rural communities, main offices were distant and remote;
- Local people had little or no influence over service patterns and provision;
- There was little evidence of joint planning;
- There was no recognition of local needs;
- 'We do not know who does what'.

Everyone wanted something that was local, belonged to the community and provided a unified service. So was born the concept of the 'One Stop Shop'. The area of Wheatley Hill and Thornley was chosen to pilot an initiative and a development group set up. Its members included a Nurse Manager, Social Services Team Manager and the Health Authority Locality Director. This group identified an existing health clinic as an appropriate 'shop' and supported by joint finance arranged its refurbishment. Discussions with local agencies produced a sessional programme offering a range of services and activities. As a focus for health care the 'One Stop Shop' provides children's services, good parenting skills training, ophthalmology, audiometrics, a diabetic clinic and chiropody. Weekly sessions are provided by the DSS Benefits Agency, Probation, Housing Welfare and local support groups. The centre is used for child care access visits and is a practice base for district nurses, community psychiatric nurses and care managers from the Older Persons and Mental Health Teams. The facility continues to develop and is now a venue for the weekly Primary Care Team meeting. This initiative has enabled staff to promote shared information systems and they are currently examining the possibility of establishing jointly held records. There is demonstrably a greater level of understanding of individual agency roles and responsibilities. Most important, the centre is highly regarded by local people who have a strong sense of ownership and commitment to its continuing success. They value the co-ordinated, inter-agency response to their unique needs and the real voice it offers in the joint care planning framework.

Primary care team development

A second development in Easington District which also began in 1994 focused specifically on Primary Care Team working arrangements. There are 18 GP practices across the District the quality of whose relationships with Social Services varied from good to non-existent. The Older Persons team decided to align care managers to each practice whilst retaining a central team location. Each practice knows its Care Manager and there are regular meetings between staff. Frequently the interface between Social Services and Primary Care Team is described as a black hole typified by misunderstanding and mistrust. The pattern of alignment is built on the principle that if people know each other, meet regularly and talk together they are more likely to work together effectively. Team members have established a clearer understanding of each other's responsibilities and constraints. Communication is much improved. These enhanced Primary Care Teams are initiating systems to provide joint assessments for older people which are already routine to all over-85s. They are developing links with secondary health care providers to supply patient profiles at the point of hospital admission which contribute to therapeutic interventions and facilitate good quality discharge planning. Again, they provide a vehicle for information and opinion to the JCB and so help shape services within the locality.

JOINT COMMISSIONING WITH PRIMARY CARE

The Joint Commissioning Project (JCP) was an initiative based in the south of the County. Although it ended as a project in 1995 it has been instrumental in influencing agency thinking on primary care working arrangements and has provided a valuable source of information to colleagues not only within County Durham but also in other areas of the Country.

JCP originated in 1992 as a joint venture between County Durham Social Services Department, the County Durham Health Authority, the Northern Regional Health Authority and two GP fundholding practices. It was funded by the Regional Health Authority and sought to inform community care thinking and explore the potential of operational joint commissioning. A full time care manager was based at each GP practice as an integrated member of the Primary Care Team. Their work, and the project as a whole were managed by a Project Manager. As older people are recognised as the largest users of health and social care resources the remit was to design a coordinated care management approach to the health and social care needs of the over-75s. The original aims were:

- To promote the provision of more appropriate and efficient service arrangements which are well integrated and coordinated and tailored to individual need;
- To establish mechanisms for the joint commissioning of social and health care services for people aged 75 and over;
- To investigate user and carer perceptions of social and health care needs and the priorities awarded to those needs;
- To promote the lessons learnt in County Durham and the Northern Health Authority Region.

Between June 1993 and December 1994 the JCP was subject to a formative evaluation by the Nuffield Institute for Health. The project was fortunate to have a flexible, evolutionary remit which could be shaped by the evaluation and, most importantly, through an experiential process. Without this responsiveness the JCP would have been rigid and inhibited. During the first 6 months of the project a number of key issues emerged and were addressed. As explained below, these have relevance to all aspects of joint working and were not unique to the JCP.

The team members and Steering Group talked together readily and easily but came to recognise that it was not, necessarily, the same language. An early finding from the evaluation showed a lack of clarity and understanding of the original aims. Each agency partner had, for example, a different perception of joint commissioning, care management and care planning. Each worked from a different agenda. Once the problem was recognised it became relatively easy to revise the objectives to reflect individual and shared expectations. The following new objectives were concrete, measurable and gave a clearer sense of direction:

- To identify the core activities of joint commissioning in GP fundholding practices;
- To establish links with staff outside of the JCP to enable comparisons to be made;
- To define the potential for health and social care gains;
- To examine the most cost effective ways of delivering services in line with identified need;
- To determine the most effective ratio of care manager time per patient numbers in relation to people aged 65 years and over;
- To identify the benefits and resource implications of developing shared information systems, both manual and computerised, between agencies;
- To identify the health and social care needs focusing around the Primary Care Team to explore future work force planning requirements.

The second major issue was that of trust and understanding. There is a well documented history of poor working relationships between GPs/Primary Care Teams and Social Services Departments based upon stereo-typical imagery. It was necessary for the team to share these perceptions openly to acknowledge how they had arisen and then 'put them to bed'. Inevitably the question of confidentiality arose. The team agreed from the beginning that there should be full access to each other's records and information systems recognising the integrity of the professional partnership. Therefore, confidentiality was never allowed to become a 'problem' or an insurmountable issue. By the end of the project the practices' and

Social Services' computerised databases had been linked electronically giving full access, one to the other.

If the Primary Care Team was to successfully undertake its new role a corporate approach became essential to understand the principles and process of Care Management. The Project Manager arranged and delivered training sessions which evolved into ongoing mutually educative relationships. A model emerged whereby the most appropriate member of the team, GP Community Nurse or Care Manager accepted the lead role and coordinated other input into the assessment and care planning processes. The project did not quite achieve the goal of allocating each other's resources. However, whichever team member led the assessment, that judgement of needs was accepted by the whole team at the care planning stage. Therefore the Community Nurse could request home care without the care manager making a separate assessment, the care manager could request referral for rehabilitation without question demonstrating inter-agency trust and cooperation.

Finally, it was necessary to consider traditionally held power bases and demonstrate a willingness to relinquish certain controls. This concept was succinctly described by one GP as: 'If the Care Manager asks me to jump I ask, how high?' This model of integrated team working should not be seen by anyone as an opportunity to offload the more problematic patients onto another colleague or agency. The presence of the care manager did not reduce any other team member's workload and on occasions almost certainly increased it. What it did provide was the opportunity to make the best use of the different skill mix of the team. Social care matters highlighted by the GP could be directed to the care manager for resolution. In turn the care manager was able to access immediate medical or nursing interventions. This approach allowed the team to provide a coordinated response to crisis intervention and a corporate view on risk management. A Project initiated welfare rights campaign acknowledged the link between poverty, ill health and social deprivation. £260 000 additional benefits over 1 year were accessed for local people.

A Primary Care-led joint service

A number of key lessons were identified during the evaluation of the JCP and they provide a useful framework for Primary Care-led joint working. The likelihood of information being shared is clearly enhanced by the proximity of primary care and social services staff.

Accurate and readily available shared information is essential to the quality of assessment and care planning which in turn can determine appropriate agency responsibility. The evaluation highlighted that the speed of response was considerably greater in the JCP than in comparison with traditional, centralised agency services and priority was jointly determined. There is evidence that the JCP Primary Care Teams were more able to reconcile the wishes of users and carers through an holistic approach to their joint needs. As case monitoring was a corporate responsibility JCP care managers learned about changes in need at an early stage and had greater opportunities for preventive work based on earlier intervention. The JCP care managers each carried an average caseload of 60 people in the various stages of assessment and care planning or whose circumstances were extremely volatile and unstable. At any given time approximately 100 more people in each practice were monitored under care management systems by other Primary Care Team members.

The JCP model provided a single entry point for accessing health and social services which was alert and responsive to local circumstances. Service users and their carers appreciated the accessibility of staff and were grateful for the lack of duplication and repetition from the team. Continuity of care was provided during hospitalisation when the care manager acted as the contact point between the hospital and the Primary Care Team. There is evidence to suggest that within the JCP hospital discharges were better planned and coordinated resulting in fewer readmissions. A measure of the added value brought to primary care working through care manager attachment is proved by the commitment of each agency to secure funding for the arrangement to continue after the project ended.

FUTURE CHALLENGES

While these examples all demonstrate the successful implementation of local schemes it would be misleading to ignore the occasional failures Durham has experienced and lessons must be drawn from them. There are a number of factors common to those schemes that have tried yet failed. These include:

- Inadequate preparation. Successful schemes require the investment of time, energy and ongoing management support. Protocols and shared understanding are important and *joint working does not just happen by chance*;

- The partners in the scheme must be willing, it cannot be imposed upon them;
- There must be open and robust communication channels within the Primary Care Team which allow differences arising from individual professional perspectives to be considered, acknowledged and respected;
- Whether aligned or attached to Primary Care Teams, care managers must have access to other team members as required. There must be an opportunity to discuss individual patients and to share information;
- There must be willingness to work jointly and not offload work inappropriately to other colleagues. This includes a commitment to joint assessment and care planning, consensus decision making and corporate risk management.

Each organisation operates within its own legal, cultural and financial systems. Joint commissioning provides a means of tackling the barriers which are created by this diversity. At the strategic level it is a joint commitment between agencies which leads to the identification of shared responsibilities and objectives. Agencies work together to coordinate their purchasing capacity and address shortfalls in service provision. As a process which translates joint planning into joint action it must avoid unwieldy bureaucratic mechanisms if it is to be responsive to the needs of individuals.

At an operational level, joint commissioning represents the co-ordination of the care of individuals across health and social care boundaries. Staff are encouraged and supported in developing practices which overcome organisational divides. Response is based upon the needs of the individual and is not determined by whichever agency is first contacted. The most effective models for joint working are those which evolve gradually taking account of local factors and which allow for individual preferred working patterns and practices. Joint working should seek to accommodate preference within a mutually acceptable framework. The benefits of an integrated operational joint commissioning approach include the facility for joint care packages and joint care management. It provides a responsive service to those in crisis and offers alternatives to hospital admission or institutional care whenever possible. Good quality hospital discharges are maintained by ensuring available community support networks are in place.

A Durham-style joint Primary Care Strategy is a model which

can address the challenges in health and social care for the next decade and beyond. However, it does not just happen spontaneously; there must be a sharing of vision, commitment and resources to unlock the potential to turn the concept of a primary care led service into a reality.

Part Three: The Response

8. The Communications Challenge: It's good to talk ... and be heard!

Valerie Iles

Conflict of culture and communication have been conventionally regarded as virtually a chronic condition in respect of the relationship between Health and Social Services. The advent of general management over the past decade has done disappointingly little to challenge this convention, given its essentially internal focus on organisational change. In setting the scene for Part Three of this book, and paving the way for a series of practice-based contributions which highlight how the different dimensions of effectiveness can be positively put together by Health and Social Services in primary care, Valerie Iles picks up this challenge. The following chapter is an account of sound, evidence-based management frameworks for understanding and improving cross-boundary communication, and for recognising, respecting and reconciling cultural differences. They are an objective, neutral and usable methodology and, if applied in the right spirit, start to suggest that there may yet be an affirmative answer to the book's question.

FRAMEWORKS

All politically correct definitions of health include a social dimension. Much lip service is paid, for example, to the World Health Organisation's definition: 'health is a state of complete physical, mental and social well-being and not merely the absence of disease and infirmity'. No-one disputes the link between housing, education, employment status and health; an argument rages over whether poor health causes social disadvantage or vice versa, but everyone agrees that social and health inequalities coincide. And yet all too rarely are health or social problems tackled in a genuinely holistic manner, across the health and social services divide. Why is this? Is it because of the organisational boundaries that have to be crossed? Or, as suggested in Chapter 1, are other more fundamental, more intractable causes involved? Exploring the effectiveness of communication between different professionals may help us to answer this question.

Listen to social workers describing their interactions with GPs; the complaints of never being allowed to finish a sentence, of being pushed to come up with a ready solution to a convincingly diagnosed but unidimensional problem. Or the reverse: GPs letting off steam about woolly thinking social workers with verbal diarrhoea who do not understand the meaning of the word 'urgent' and always want to complicate matters by bringing in extraneous unrelated factors. Aspects of this stereotype are so widespread that we should not blame individuals for their failure to communicate; we must look elsewhere. Should we look at organisational boundaries? Or are other forces at work?

There are a number of reasons why, in particular, inter-professional communication is bound to be difficult, regardless of organisational context. Some are to do with the *task* the professions undertake, some with the *manner* in which it is undertaken, some with the causes of *status* within and between professions, and some with the two distinct *roles* all professionals are required to play. This chapter discusses these obstacles to effective inter-disciplinary working and explores ways in which they can be addressed in primary care.

THE TASK OF HEALTH AND SOCIAL CARE PROFESSIONALS

Let us take as a working definition of health and social care: 'work which enables development of the potentials of clients'[1] and the role of the relevant professionals as 'diagnosing obstacles to the development of potentials and intervening to address the obstacles with which they are best qualified to deal'.[2] The obstacles to the development of potentials can be many and varied and they can occur at any or many of the levels included in the hierarchy below.[3]

level +2	patient's community
level +1	patient's family
level 0	patient as a whole
level −1	major patient part e.g. chest, abdomen, head
level −2	physiological system: e.g. cardiovascular system, respiratory system

level –3	system part or organ: e.g. heart, major vessels, lungs
level –4	organ part or tissue: e.g. myocardium, bone marrow
level –5	cell: e.g. epithelial cell, fibroblast, lymphocyte
level –6	cell part e.g. cell membrane, organelles, nucleus
level –7	macromolecule: e.g. enzyme, structural protein, nucleic acid
level –8	micromolecule: e.g. glucose, ascorbic acid
level –9	atoms or ions: e.g. sodium ion

This is a hierarchy because objects from each level in it comprise a combination of elements at the next lowest level. For example molecules are made up of atoms; families are made up of *individuals*. Thus the health of an individual or family can be described at a number of different levels in this hierarchy (or 'knowledge network'); in terms of their blood electrolyte levels, their heart function, their personal mobility, their relationships, their employment.

Knowledge networks of this kind demonstrate a number of known features, including the following:

- It is only possible to focus attention on one level (and those immediately above and below it) at a time. We can track up and down the levels, and with experience the speed at which we do so increases, but we cannot instantaneously focus on blood medication levels *and* the impact they may have on a patient's family relationships.
- At each level we need a different level of language. If we use a lower level language at a higher level it is over descriptive and tedious without adding anything. Describing the heart in terms of all of its constituent cells takes a long time and is not necessary. Conversely the use of a higher level language at a lower level results in confusion, or nonsense, because it is over-rich; it tries to ascribe attributes that do not emerge until higher levels to lower level items. For example, colour has no meaning at molecular level, neither does sentience at the level of cells or of organs.
- Numbers are often useful at lower levels (blood electrolyte levels for example). They enable expression of a degree of abnormality and a measure of whether things are getting better or worse. At higher levels quantification is more difficult. Where high level descriptions are converted to numbers (e.g. *Activities for Daily Living scores*) they should be used with great care since they are

attempting to represent a rich, ambiguous, fuzzy, multi-faceted reality. Just as words need to be used differently at different levels so do numbers. We cannot manipulate numbers referring to high levels in the same way as those at lower levels.

- As we ascend the levels individuality increases and uniformity decreases. One electron looks very much like any other electron and is readily distinguished from a neutron or proton. The distinction between (and classification of) one set of family relationships and another is not so straightforward.
- To solve any problems expert consideration of all levels will be necessary.

Different professions tend to have expertise at different levels; indeed many of the health care professions emerged as knowledge of the different levels developed. Within professions too, different disciplines focus on different levels; so although the medical profession as a whole includes those with expertise at levels-1 to -9, hospital based consultants concentrate on levels lower than their colleagues in general practice. This leads almost inevitably to problems of communication, to issues of status, and to reliance on different kinds of evidence on which to base decisions.

Status differentials arise out of a number of factors but one of these is the 'hardness' or definitiveness of the knowledge base deployed. In this knowledge network it is the lower levels that are more definitive, descriptions at higher levels are more ambiguous and more dependent on context. Status will be explored more fully later in this chapter, but already we can see that we cannot increase the status of a given group of professionals, or decrease that of another, simply by declaration.

Communication problems arise because of the different levels of language required at the different levels. Some communication problems can be overcome if practitioners explain their 'tracking' through the levels, recognising that such explanations can be understood even by people who do not have a complete understanding of each of the levels concerned. Others are more intractable since some groups will not be aware of the existence of the elements at lower levels, and others are unaware of the complexity of ambiguity at higher ones.

Now that there is such pressure to base decisions on evidence it is important to draw on evidence that is relevant. At lower levels their definitive nature allows precise questions and answers. To the question: 'Does a drug a have an effect on blood glucose and by how much?' the answers can be: yes, no, x.75%. Anything less precise may well be an example of woolly thinking.

At higher levels the fuzziness between boundaries permits only qualified answers unless the questions are unimaginably complex. So to a question: 'Does community care provide better outcomes for people with long term mental illness?' the correct, accurate answer will be: maybe: sometimes; in conditions x, y and z we found ... These answers are no more woolly than those of yes or no to the first question. Indeed a 'precise' answer of yes or no *would* be sloppy thinking.

This difference in question and in answer requires different ways of gathering evidence, the Randomised Controlled Trial being wholly appropriate to the first and not to the second; the second relying on more qualitative methods. Unless different professions understand and value the differences in research methods required and the reasons for them we will perpetuate unhelpful stereotypes and poor communication.

THE MANNER OF UNDERTAKING CARE TASKS

In health and social services the use and transfer of information are the essence of the task. Eliciting and conveying information are critical and in primary care this usually takes place through conversation. We converse using rituals which we have developed in response to our circumstances, most often adopting the rituals of role models. Often these rituals are not apparent to us and indeed when conversing with someone using the same ritual we experience no difficulty in understanding nor in being understood. When we try to exchange information with someone adopting a different ritual however, we distort each other's meaning.

Deborah Tannen[4] has identified a number of these rituals. Her research and the research on which she draws suggests a correlation between different rituals and different genders. She has not looked at differences between professions or between personality types, both of which may prove interesting and just as, or more, useful; however if we take her conclusions and look simply at the gender of the role models in the professions comprising health and social care, we may imagine that the rituals adopted by those professions will not all be the same.

Tannen's research suggests that the conversational rituals common among men include: using opposition such as banter, joking, teasing and playful put-downs; and expending effort to avoid the one-down position in an interaction. Men will present their own ideas in a certain and absolute form and wait to see if they are challenged in a similarly forceful manner. They can argue heatedly with each other and then unlock horns and be as friendly as before. Rituals common among women involve finding ways of maintaining an appearance of equality, taking into account the effect of the exchange on the other person, expending effort to down-play the speaker's authority.

Women are much more likely than men to ask questions if they need to know the answer; to say 'I'm sorry' when they are not apologising but sympathising; to thank, expecting to trigger an inkind response; and to offer compliments. They are also more inclined to engage in 'troubles-talk' in which they complain about a situation in order not to have a problem solved, but to prompt a similar complaint thus developing some solidarity. Men are likely to be more direct in their requests or instructions than are women.

Tannen stresses that other cultural influences contribute to the development of these conversational rituals and that within gender differences can be as great as those between genders. Her point is that we need to be aware of our own conversational rituals and those of others if we are to communicate effectively. She says 'Talking, like walking, it is something we do without stopping to question how we are doing it. But we must.'

The different professions providing health and social services have developed different conversational rituals and will fail to collaborate optimally unless they recognise these and plan their conversational strategies.

STATUS DIFFERENTIALS WITHIN AND BETWEEN PROFESSIONS

Many a post-event debrief about a multi-disciplinary case-conference exposes tensions which have their root in feelings about status. If care decisions are to be informed by the practitioners with the most relevant expertise then they must not be inhibited from providing that expertise by perceptions of inequality of status.

We have already seen that in the world at large status is conferred on individuals and groups dealing in hard, technical knowledge-bases and less so on those involved with 'softer' subjects. In part this is to do with economics; it takes a long time and large intellectual capacity to get to grips with the knowledge base of medicine or law. Individuals with this knowledge are therefore scarce and scarcity confers status. But it is not only the technicality of the knowledge base that is important because if it is entirely logical it can be replaced by computers or parcelled up into smaller tasks and given to people with less expensive training. The ratio of technicality to 'indeterminacy'[5] is important. In other words, there must also be a significant interpretive function if the profession is to enjoy high status.

Status cannot therefore be awarded or claimed by individuals or groups but arises out of economic and cultural forces in society at large. It will therefore be unaffected by changes to organisational boundaries or funding streams. Where differentials are unhelpful, and in the provision of holistic care they are unhelpful, then they must be explored and understood and efforts made to ensure that information arising from different sources is weighted according to relevance and not to the status of the provider.

One way of protecting individuals from inappropriate use of 'clout' by higher status colleagues is to put the weight of a separate organisation and its hierarchy behind them. Organisational boundaries therefore address a need and if they are to be removed an alternative way must be found for that need to be addressed.

THE TWO DISTINCT ROLES REQUIRED OF PROFESSIONALS

In every society, suggests social anthropologist Jane Jacobs,[6] there is a need for two distinct roles: the guardianship of land and other resources; and the trading of goods and services. Jacobs' research also indicates that these roles are associated with particular sets (or syndromes) of behaviours and that these syndromes must be employed, entire and uncorrupted by behaviours associated with the other role, whenever a role is undertaken. Before we consider the relevance for providers of health and social services let us explore Jacobs' ideas.

By looking at evidence of which behaviours are esteemed and in which circumstances, and also which behaviours are disparaged and when, Jacobs was able to draw up three lists. The first is a list of behaviours that are universally esteemed regardless of context. This includes responsibility, cooperation, courage, moderation, mercy, common-sense, foresight, judgement, competence, perseverance, faith, energy, patience and wisdom.

The other two lists are the behaviours associated with the two roles. When engaging in a trading role we are encouraged to shun force and come to voluntary agreement, to be honest, to collaborate easily with strangers, to compete with other traders, to respect contracts, use initiative and enterprise, be open to inventiveness and novelty, be efficient, promote comfort and convenience, dissent honestly for the sake of the task, and be optimistic that by taking action we can influence our fortunes. Jacobs points out that historically trading took place in cities, that the word cosmopolitan (from the Greek meaning universal people) referred to the city practices of dealing easily with people from other countries and cultures; that serfs referred to the 'free air of the city', meaning that there they had the same rights as any one else because their rights were gained through contacts and not through feudal hierarchy.

In contrast, people in guardianship roles frown on people who trade ('new money' versus 'old money'), they exert prowess (using force where necessary to require obedience to laws), insist on obedience and discipline, adhere to (and venerate) tradition, require loyalty, take vengeance, deceive for the sake of the task (spying for example), dispense largesse, (distributing wealth, power etc.), are exclusive (is he one of 'us'?), show fortitude, exhibit fatalism, and treasure honour (and 'face').

We can easily see that in society we need an active commercial sector adopting the trading role and behaviours **and** a wise government undertaking the guardianship role and its behaviours. Jacobs' research suggests however that the roles and behaviours must not be mixed together, if they become so then a 'monstrous hybrid' develops. She cites concentration camps as an example of such a hybrid — a mix of industrious efficiency with deceit, exclusiveness, vengeance. If trading behaviours are introduced into the guardianship role, or vice versa, then virtues become vices. In order to prevent this happening there are only two ways of keeping the roles distinct. One is a caste system, in which individuals permanently reside in one role or the other. The second, more morally defensible one, is a system of 'knowledgeable flexibility' in which people move knowingly from one role to another, selecting the appropriate behaviours as they move.

Jacobs also observes that individuals and groups often have a cast of mind rooted in one of these syndromes of behaviours and will espouse those behaviours as virtues, regardless of the context and of the role properly to be played.

What is the relevance of this to the provision of health and social services in primary care? First, many professionals are required to undertake both trading and guardianship roles and slip, unawares, from one to the other experiencing tension and dilemma as they then apply inappropriate behaviours. This tension will not bode well for self-esteem and collaborative interaction, and the decisions reached (and actions taken) will not be optimal for either patient or society.

Second, the different professions may have different casts of mind, and thus pursue different behavioural norms, castigating others for failing to adopt their preferred syndrome. If we are to have effective collaboration and effective decision-making we must therefore increase knowledge within and between the professions of these two roles, of the trading nature of the interaction with an individual client and the guardianship role relating to use of resources, of the behaviours which need to be associated with them. Perhaps too, we should question the development of systems in which people are required to move from one role to another on a frequent basis. But that may be heresy to proponents of the Primary Care-Led NHS!

EFFECTIVE COMBINATIONS OF HEALTH AND SOCIAL SERVICES

There are, as we have seen, a number of reasons why providers of health and social services will find it difficult to work together. There are many others including, for example, the phenomenon known as Group Think and differences in ethical paradigms. These arise as a result of the nature of the care task and care roles, early developmental influences, and economic and sociological factors. None of these will be affected by the bringing together of health and social services in primary care. If this initiative is to be successful it will be necessary to address these issues explicitly. Organisational merger in the absence of so doing will not lead to effective collaboration and holistic care.

Promoting a trans-care culture of generosity and of discipline is the way this can be achieved. As this must replace cultures of jealousy and self-righteous helplessness this will take time and concerted effort. It will require of all concerned a shift from a concentration on policy 'whats' to systemic 'hows'.

Generosity and discipline can be described as follows:

Generosity

There are five elements of generosity:
1. *Choosing to care.*
   Engaging in acts of work and/or courage to nurture the growth

of organisation members and clients, and to remove obstacles to the enablement of potential.
2. *Choosing to expect the best of others.*
Investing energy in an accurate assessment of what is their best, making expectations clear, and constructively challenging suboptimal performance or behaviour.
3. *Choosing to meet hostility, aggression or arrogance with compassion.*
Identifying the cause of the fear that lies behind this behaviour and using intellect and empathy rather than anger to engage with them and their arguments.
4. *Choosing to include and value rather than exclude and compare.*
Seeking the contributions that others can make and delighting in their value instead of indulging in self-righteous triumphalism at their mistakes or limitations.
5. Underpinning our ability to exhibit generosity in these ways is our *choosing to fashion own self-image and not allow it to be shaped by the ungenerous.* This involves identifying a realistic self-image based on contribution (making a difference) rather than achievement (acquiring a reputation); aiming at satisfaction (progress towards personal mission) rather than enjoyment (responding to motivational goals); and seeking evidence of progress towards goals. This evidence will not include the distorted perceptions of the ungenerous.

Discipline

There are four elements of discipline (described by Scott Peck in *The Road Less Travelled*)[7]

1. *Acceptance of responsibility.*
Realising that 'If I have a problem then it is my problem and it is up to me to solve it. If I am not part of its solution then I am part of the problem.' Blaming other people, circumstances or situations places the blamer in 'victim' mode, choosing to feel helpless and often self-righteous. This is a failure to accept responsibility. Acceptance of responsibility includes careful analysis of the problem, identification of obstacles to its resolution and deployment of resources (often the time required to frame *persuasive* collaborative arguments) with the genuine aim of overcoming those obstacles.
2. *Dedication to reality.*
Working hard to allow our model of the world to be as close to reality as possible, thus increasing the validity and wisdom of

our choices and decisions. Our models include perceptions of other people and of ourselves, and we must constantly challenge those perceptions and allow constructive challenge from others.
3. *Delaying of gratification.*
Scheduling difficult activities before more pleasurable ones so that we maximise our contribution and experience pleasure with greater enjoyment. This requires us to see that our time is us; if we waste time we are wasting something precious. It is easy to see that if we have a list of tasks for the day and some cause us anxiety or even pain and we expect to enjoy others, then delaying gratification would require us to undertake the unpleasant ones first. It is harder to see that giving enough time to the solving of a problem (and not, for example, jumping to a solution that does not work and then giving up) is another form of this principle.
4. *Balancing.*
Exercising judgement about when to accept responsibility, to accept and when to hold others to the proper acceptance of it as theirs; when to challenge perceptions and when to withhold some truth; when to delay a pleasurable activity and when to enjoy oneself. This requires difficult decisions on an ongoing basis.

If we are to engender a culture of generosity and discipline then we must examine carefully all the elements of the care system for aspects which do not allow it to flourish. In particular we must 'drive out fear'[8] since fear is a major inhibitor of Generosity and Discipline at both personal and organisational levels. For effective combinations of health and social services in primary care especially, this must entail a review of professional educational and formative socialisation processes as well as of systems of supervision, and accountability. It will also require means of convincing all health and social care providers that they are not innocent bystanders, observing situations over which they have little influence, but that they are active players in a dynamic system which they must inevitably influence. Further, that the outcome of that system (client health and wellbeing) depends crucially upon them and their relationships with other elements of the system, whether or not they are brought together under one organisational roof.

REFERENCES

1. Seedhouse J 1991 Liberating Medicine. John Wiley & Sons, New York
2. Ibid

3. Blois M 1984 Information & Medicine. University of California Press, Berkeley
4. Tannen D 1995, Talking 9 to 5. Virago, London
5. Turner B 1995 Medical Power and Social Knowledge. Sage Publications, London
6. Jacobs J 1994 Systems of Survival. Hodder and Stoughton, London
7. Peck MS 1979 The Road Less Travelled. Arrow, New York
8. Driving out fear is a tenet of EW Deming, described for example in Walton M Deming Management at Work. Mercury Books, London

9. Professional Effectiveness: The Somerset example

Heather Roughton

The willingness in Somerset of both the local NHS and Social Services Department to behave as if one 'learning organisation' is a beautiful illustration of the kind of management generosity and discipline Valerie Iles describes in the previous chapter as the essential prerequisites of effective combinations — in primary care as in any other service sector. The non-territorial approach to the concept of evaluation captures this generosity, and the automatic application of research findings to joint training programmes exemplifies the disciplined approach to development. Somerset is one of those areas which seems to provide a role model to the rest of us and the importance of building up a joint history is well illustrated by the lessons learnt together from the experience of working together over the past decade to close and replace long stay institutions for people with mental illness and learning disabilities.

THE SOMERSET STYLE

Joint research is only one aspect of the joint partnership between Health and Social Services in Somerset and its distinctive approach to Community Care. It is based on the understanding that working together achieves more than the same level of effort, resources and expenditure applied separately, a view which predates but reflects the concept of 'joint commissioning'. As will be seen it also requires a rigorous approach to defining the 'core business' of each partner.

In this paper the term 'Research' is used as a generic description for a variety of activities: studies designed to investigate the extent of need in target populations, the monitoring and evaluation of innovations in service arrangements, the evaluation of outcomes, and audits of performance. These variously contributed to the way in which the county implemented the recent Community Care reforms.

PRIMARY AND COMMUNITY CARE

In Somerset discussions about the changes required by the Community Care legislation began early in 1991. They quickly established that a comprehensive assessment of individuals with complex needs should be available from a multidisciplinary team, and a cross-agency group of practitioners was formed to work on the details, including a common assessment format. Multidisciplinary teams are an established way of working in hospital settings, but in the community the various professionals who may contribute to assessments work in different organisations, and in different locations. The Somerset model of specialist teams for different client groups is common in many local authorities, and has enabled social services staff to be more effective in many respects. However it makes coordination with primary health care teams, which are generic in character, more difficult.

In the new arrangements social services staff and local primary care teams need to develop a common understanding of the priorities for the care needs of the people they work with and coordinate care plans. Examination of existing links revealed regular contact between health and social services in Somerset, with about 40% of referrals to social services coming from health staff. This provided evidence that a high proportion of the most vulnerable people in the community were already known to both health and social care staff.

Since referrals were most frequently channelled through the district nurse, even when the GP prompted the request, it seemed that GPs were not the key figures in inter-professional communication. They have a vital role in identifying individuals who need additional support, and should 'trigger' the assessment process. GPs contribute their view of what medical problems the individual is currently experiencing, how this might progress, and the implications of planned medical interventions.

There was also a pragmatic reason for adopting this approach in a period of considerable upheaval for health care. In 1991 all acute and community services in Somerset were in the first wave of NHS Trusts and, in addition, the first pilots in fundholding practices were being developed. It was then felt that GPs would have little appetite for taking on heavier responsibilities in social care as well as coping with these changes. A more general assumption at the time was that they had neither the time nor the knowledge base for coordinating and managing complex care arrangements.

Nurse assessors

The conclusion was that responsibility for working with social services local teams to carry out assessment, and developing care plans should rest with district nurses and community psychiatric nurses (CPNs). At the request of the Health Authority, the NHS Trusts carried out an audit of the effectiveness of district nurse assessments. The result was that G-grade nurses became designated Nurse Assessors. Assessors became team leaders. The Health Authority in Somerset used development funds to enhance community nursing services to support the nurse assessor arrangements, thus encouraging the Trusts to review the skill-mix of their teams.

In assessing people who need community care provision, social workers and occupational therapists routinely enquire about health factors. When they identify any concerns relating to health, the nurse assessor is invited to contribute a more detailed assessment. The role of the nurse assessor is not confined to assessment. The assessors jointly agree on the care arrangements with the user and carer, and if the care has a predominantly health/nursing care component, nurses also continue to monitor and review care arrangements, i.e. they act as care managers. This includes all placements made with public funding in nursing homes.

Nursing home proprietors have welcomed this arrangement which ensures a professional nursing input into monitoring the care they provide. It has also given community nurses an opportunity to enhance the quality of care, by informal support, updating and guidance. Training on the role of Inspection and Registration Officers encourages them to communicate concerns about standards of care.

Preparing together

In the months prior to implementation of the reforms, a county-wide training programme was established, designed to develop effective joint working, and understanding of the assessment and care management arrangements. The training was jointly funded and devised by an inter-agency group. When the reforms were introduced in 1993, assessors in local teams and acute hospitals had undertaken 5 days of joint training.

All participants completed an evaluation of the training programme, as well as suggestions for future training requirements. These were analysed to inform the next stage of the joint training strategy, which is now coordinated by a trainer, funded through Joint Finance.

A lunch-time presentation at venues throughout the county informed GPs and practice managers of the proposed changes.

DEVOLVED BUDGETS AND LOCAL RESPONSIBILITIES

The Social Services Department has devolved budgets to local teams so that the staff directly involved with the individual and their family in the assessment phase decide on the appropriate care. In each area, social services managers hold a single purchasing budget, comprising the earmarked Community Care funding made available by the government (the Special Transitional Grant) together with the 'mainstream' budget allocation for their client group. Each manager has an indicative allocation for residential and domiciliary care for the relevant client group, but is able to use the total budget flexibly, to meet needs appropriately for the individual, rather than fitting people into resources.

Part of the Social Services budget is identified to support those people with nursing care needs as well as those needing social care, and is 'ring-fenced'. Responsibility for this is shared with local nurse managers in the NHS Trusts who also have an annual indicative amount to cover anticipated levels of nursing home placements for the most dependent people.

Nurse managers liaise with their SSD colleagues locally on a day-to-day basis to agree on admissions to nursing homes, and complex care arrangements. The arrangements mean that at local level, health and social services managers have a shared commitment to managing costs and demand, and achieving the most effective care within resources. Disagreements about the identified needs inevitably occur but are resolved locally. The trust and cooperation which was required between the authorities in setting up the arrangements has thus been translated to local operational levels. Dialogue replaces confrontation, and staff who are faced with pressures on local resources tackle this as a shared problem, and endeavour to find shared solutions. This in turn has led staff to develop joint initiatives to address gaps in local provision.

Access to the 'nursing care' budget is available on the basis of agreed care plans following joint assessment — either to fund a nursing home admission *or to provide the additional nursing care in the community for people who would otherwise be in a nursing home*. A 'perverse incentive' can exist for primary health care to promote admission to a nursing home when their time and budget is under pressure, and the full cost of the placement is borne by the local authority. The Somerset budgetary arrangements minimise this prospect. Senior officers monitor the commissioning budgets to ensure that Social Services money is not substituting for the agreed level of nursing care to be provided through the Health Authority contracts with the Trusts.

Undetected or untreated health problems can be significant factors in avoidable and costly admission to residential units. Timely diagnosis, treatment, and rehabilitation should diminish the need for long-term care, and the involvement of the nurse assessor ensures that health care issues are addressed at an early stage of potential admissions.

Joint criteria serve to guide staff in deciding whether a nursing home or residential home is appropriate. It is therefore agreed that a nursing home placement is appropriate when an individual has significant nursing needs on a 24-hour basis or at unpredictable intervals, which could not be met by community nurses visiting them in another setting, either their own home or a residential care home.

There is a clear understanding in Somerset that nursing homes should deliver a different level of care from residential homes, and this is reflected in the fee differential. This resulted from a study completed shortly before the Community Care reforms, which examined the dependency of residents in different settings — from specialised sheltered housing to long-stay wards. It showed that each care setting was catering for a different level of dependency with the most dependent populations being in nursing homes and long-stay wards.

Budget flexibility also helps to ensure that care needs are addressed in the setting most appropriate to the individual and their carer. It has enabled a proportion of people to be 'diverted' from nursing home care, where the effect is cost-neutral. An increasing number of extremely dependent people remain where they and their families wish them to be — at home, using the available money to purchase flexible creative care arrangements. A few have left nursing homes to return to the community. The discharge of patients from hospital has been maintained without an increase in bed-blocking.

PARTNERSHIPS IN PURCHASING AND PROVIDING

Somerset Social Services have adopted a pragmatic approach to the separation of purchasing/providing. Arrangements reflect the pace at which different services have developed in the county, and how the joint partnership with health has evolved. In the same way that GPs remain important providers of services in their own right, having a primary diagnostic/assessment role as well as a growing purchasing function, so other front-line staff (social workers, occupational therapists, and community nurses) are seen to be both providers and purchasers.

Almost all social care services for elderly people are provided in the county by the independent sector. Somerset County Council transferred all of its 26 homes for older people to an independent company in 1991 and is the only local authority to have no direct involvement in the Home Care service — which was also transferred to the independent company. Contracts to provide home care are now in operation with 14 independent organisations, and assessors of elderly people purchase care from a variety of providers.

Care for people who are mentally ill has hitherto been based on a medical model, and comprehensive health care facilities. Although this is increasingly challenged by those who use psychiatric services, only 6% of the Social Services Department's budget is spent on mental health services. The annual Mental Illness Specific Grant has enabled the local authority to develop its social care provision for those leaving hospital.

The philosophy of services for younger adults with physical disability has also been to move away from medical models of care, and to provide opportunities for them to access a wide range of facilities in the community. Hence the role of the Social Services is to support the efforts of disabled people to secure the care they need, while maintaining only a small amount of residential and day care.

However, for people with learning disabilities in Somerset the local authority is the main provider of care. These arrangements were planned in the mid-1980s when the Department of Health and Social Security launched its 'Care in the Community' action research initiative. This offered funding for projects designed to move people from institutional care to the community, and was conditional on a joint commitment by both Social Services and Health Authorities.

Somerset became one of the project sites, initially with the modest objective of moving about 70 people from what were then termed mental handicap hospitals into the community. The two authorities concluded that the needs of people with learning disabilities are primarily social, not medical. Financial arrangements between Somerset Health Authority and Social Services became the basis of an agreement to transfer *all* long-stay patients to community settings, in which Social Services became responsible for their care support.

Lessons from learning disability

The Learning Disabilities Strategy was a key point in the partnership between the planning authorities. Importantly, research and monitoring were integral to the programme, evaluating the impact on the quality of life of the participants, as well as the organisational factors which determined success.

The community care proposals for other client groups were also informed by collaborative research and survey activity in the late 1980s, designed to assess need and measure service impact. Such studies took place usually at the behest of one of the strategic planning groups. Cooperation and access were readily granted, and results were shared through the joint planning team.

With the advent of the Community Care reforms, however, joint research moved on to a different level of collaboration. While other authorities were undertaking pilots in one or two localities to test their options, Somerset had already had its major collaborative pilot, the Learning Disabilities Strategy programme. The proposals for Somerset were radical, but were not intended to be incremental; from 1 April 1993 all teams whose work involved adults needing care would be affected.

The strategy had demonstrated the value of a research programme which could provide feedback and validation to staff as they tackled changes. A joint evaluation and audit programme was therefore established to monitor the implementation of Community Care. The work was carried out by a research nurse from the Health Authority, and a planning officer from Social Services (a qualified social worker) who together were responsible for developing the audit programme and methodology. They reported to the Community Care Liaison Team (CCLT), a group of senior officers in Health and Social Services responsible for coordinating the implementation phase. Another reference group was the Community Care Monitoring Group, convened by the Health Authority with senior managers from the NHS Trusts and Social Services. Both groups met monthly at the early implementation stage.

The auditors determined that the audit method should be consistent with the practice that it was monitoring, in that it would demonstrate the cycle of identifying needs, planning, monitoring, review, which was embodied in the new assessment process. It should also adhere to the following key principles for Community care which had been promoted throughout the joint training:

- It should promote participation by the users;
- It should be responsive to the needs of users;
- It should demonstrate joint working through shared professional values;
- It should ensure feedback to participants on findings.

The cooperation of staff was vital, but the audit was likely to be seen as an added pressure as they adjusted to the changes implementation was bringing about. The auditors therefore decided to commit considerable time to involving staff, explaining the purpose of the audit, and inviting them to comment on what the key areas to be studied should be. This was no mean task, involving 20 Social Services teams in 16 different locations and community nurses/CPNs in 5 NHS Trusts. In only one locality did health and social services managers fail to find a common date for the staff to meet the audit team — with hindsight this was a fair indicator of how local relationships were developing.

The event also provided an early opportunity for staff to identify concerns and to check out their understanding of the new systems. The audit team recorded all the issues raised and undertook to forward these to the inter-agency officer group after the team had an opportunity to check the accuracy of their meeting notes.

A number of key issues were identified for the audit exercise:

- Were the appropriate people being brought into the assessment process?
- Were joint assessments being undertaken?
- Were assessments needs-led rather than reflecting current service arrangements?

- Was the shared documentation adequate?
- Were other professionals contributing to assessments where appropriate?
- How were the views of users and carers taken into account?
- Were care plans documented?
- Were care arrangements more flexible and imaginative in addressing individual needs?
- What feedback was given to users and carers?
- Were arrangements in place for care managers to coordinate the care arrangements?
- Were care arrangements reviewed?

The finalised audit schedule was circulated and a schedule of visits was agreed for a case note audit to be undertaken. The first visits planned were to teams working with elderly people, since they had the highest volume of assessments and hence would complete a viable sample more quickly — in 3 months. (Complex assessment requests for younger disabled people resulted in only a handful of assessments being completed in the first 3 months.)

Assessment records were held in client files in the social services office, but the audit team followed up enquiries on individuals assessed with the relevant community nurse to clarify elements of the joint working process if this was unclear from the case notes.

As the audit report for each client group was finalised it was submitted to the inter-agency officer group (CCLT), and the Community Care Monitoring Group. The Health Authority presented a summary to the Local Medical Committee. The reports were available to the county training group highlighting areas for attention in the next stages of the joint training programme.

In the Social Services Department the service manager groups also considered the reports.

The audit team returned to each locality to give staff feedback and facilitate action plans. The audit findings were thus fed back to practices within a matter of weeks, allowing management to be reasonably confident that the new systems were working, and giving staff confidence that problems could be addressed.

THE PRIMARY CARE DEFICIT

A total of 163 assessments were scrutinised during 1993/94. Most of the people assessed were already known to the local authority and receiving help. Approximately 40% of the complex assessments undertaken involved a nurse assessor — a figure reassuringly in line with the referral analysis. Both social work and nursing staff identified joint working as a reality and were enthusiastic about improved relationships. Amendments to the joint assessment form were advised in order to improve the recording of nurses' assessments and to clarify who had continuing responsibility as care manager.

The involvement of GPs was often poorly documented in the case record, and teams confirmed the impression that they were not fully engaged in the new processes (except when they requested an emergency nursing home bed!). Managers in two areas embarked on a development programme with local GPs. They made joint visits to local practices to discuss selected cases, sharing case planning concerns as a starting point for discussion of general principles.

Of those assessed, 130 had significant problems with their physical health and functioning and 50% had mental health problems. When care arrangements at home were set up, care tasks undertaken by carers decreased and those undertaken by care professionals increased, showing that support for carers was being offered while their role was not undermined.

An independent study was commissioned to get the views of the individuals who had been assessed and their carers. This confirmed that staff were fully involving people in identifying their needs and considering their options, but showed that there was a need to improve the information provided to them. People who had been involved in moving their relative to a residential/nursing home felt (rightly) that the complex financial issues diverted attention from the emotional impact of what was happening. They wanted care managers to give them more opportunities to discuss their feelings when a placement was made.

HOSPITAL INTERFACES

The case note audit was less informative about the practice in hospital teams, mainly because Social Service Department records did not fully reflect how decisions were made. Other groups in the hospital all had their own records. Nevertheless some key issues were identified.

The Community Care Assessment was superimposed on existing discharge arrangements, and in some cases was invoked only when a placement needed to be funded. On the plus side, patients were being referred at an early stage, but in some instances before their condition had stabilised sufficiently for aftercare plans to be sensibly determined. Community care was often seen from the hospital side as affecting only a small number of patients, primarily concerning how patients who were not fit to return home could be funded in a nursing home.

Staff in the community indicated that they were seldom consulted prior to discharge. They felt that pressure to avoid beds being blocked was the dominant factor and that the full range of options on discharge was not always considered. The hospital social workers and liaison nurses felt their role was often to mediate on behalf of patients to ensure that they were given time to consider their future, and also to achieve maximum rehabilitation. Additional training workshops on discharge planning have been held for hospital staff and local teams (regrettably, few medical staff attend).

Systems have now been established for community staff to be involved in the hospital assessment if the patient is already known to them. This has introduced a slight delay in completing assessments, balanced by more speedy and effective complex care arrangements. One NHS Trust undertook a thorough reappraisal of its discharge procedures and revised its recording system.

EFFECTIVENESS IN THE ROUND

Subsequent local studies have now moved the focus from the initial assessment of individuals to the effectiveness of the care arrangements. We were particularly interested to test our assumption that we could successfully prevent a number of admissions by effective and timely care at home. Follow-up of the original cohort a year on, showed that for many individuals the arrangements at least postponed, if they could not prevent, the move to a home.

A small study was undertaken to examine coordination of care when an out-of-hours crisis occurs. The very elderly requiring intensive support and people with mental health problems were particularly vulnerable, but all the cases identified were already known to either social services or health staff. GPs undertaking weekend cover were most likely to circumvent agreed procedures to effect a nursing home placement, even though community staff could have moved in to support people at home through the emergency. Staff now establish 'contingency plans' where people are known to be at risk and local protocols are being developed, now incorporating the primary care role and contribution.

In General Practices throughout Somerset developments such as these have helped promote a new culture of information exchange. With complete HA/GP Links achieved the Somerset GP Morbidity Project has gained national attention[3] with a cross-county sample of 12 Practices supplying the detailed data and intelligence on which increasingly tight VFM commissioning decisions have to be made for health and community care.

As resources for both health and social care come under increasing pressure the joint planning relationships have to handle additional tensions, hence monitoring hospital discharges has become submerged in the monitoring of continuing care agreements. Mutual trust and understanding have to be translated into written agreements to set boundaries to the decisions that hard-pressed front-line staff make. We need to be serious about learning and managing together.

Evaluation of the effectiveness of care must be multi-dimensional to take account of the tensions that exist — an effective speedy discharge for a hospital may be the loss of dignity and choice for the patient, a welcome admission for a nursing home, financial problems for a family, an additional demand on the primary health services, and a budgetary liability for the local authority. Joint evaluation has to acknowledge that effectiveness is not a value-free concept and that community care involves decisions taken in real-life situations which defy tidy solutions.

REFERENCES

1. Renshaw J, Hampson R, Thomason C, Darton R, Judge K, Knapp M 1988 Care in the Community: The First Steps. Gower, Aldershot
2. Lankshear G, Giarchy G 1994 Community Care Review: Service User and Carer Feedback. University of Plymouth
3. See reports on the Health Services Journal's Annual Purchasers Awards. Health Services Journal 106(5530), 21 November 1996

10. Organisational Effectiveness: The Southampton example

Jill Stannard

The Southampton and South West Hampshire District within the NHS is renowned for the soundness and innovation of its organisational development. Amongst the original three Health Commissions in the country in 1992, it became the first Authority to formally define different models of primary care-led purchasing for local adoption in 1993. These may now be seen as the genesis of the 1997 primary care legislation.

It should be no surprise, therefore, that the same rigour is now being brought to the new challenge of joint commissioning with general practices in Southampton. The chapter that follows, written this time by a Social Services Department senior manager following an attachment to the local health authority, demonstrates again the importance of specifying and structuring the future organisational frameworks required for combining health and social services in primary care. Critical to these is the agreement on resourcing policy, and in particular the need to find compatible answers to the critical issue of deciding what the demographic and geographic units of financial allocations should be.

THE LOCAL TRACK RECORD

Like many Social Service Departments Hampshire has a successful record of joint commissioning with Health Authorities. Commissioning plans exist for mental health, learning disabilities and some elderly services. Strategies for closing long stay hospitals are being implemented. One of the earliest strategies (1992) involved the closure of a long stay psychiatric hospital and the setting up of locally based community mental health teams. When these teams were established the relevance of GPs was given little consideration. At the operational level a great deal of time and effort was required to help staff from a local health trust to work effectively with Social Services staff. Joint Finance was used to fund an integrated training programme focusing on team building to deliver coordinated health and social care services. 4 years later the number of fundholders has increased and a total purchasing pilot has been established. Dissatisfied with the level of care provided by the NHS Trust the GPs have changed their contract and now purchase their mental health services from a neighbouring Trust. The consequences for SSD operational staff are vast; relationships and working arrangements are having to be rebuilt with the new provider. Some have argued that this is maverick GP purchasing and is wasteful of public resources but the lesson in this is clear — joint commissioning with GPs is essential for organisational effectiveness. The question is how to do it!

The Department of Health noted in their 1993/94 community care monitoring that: *'The involvement of GPs and PHCTs in strategic commissioning i.e. at DHA/LA level, was very under developed.'*

THE FOUR PREREQUISITES FOR COMMISSIONING WITH PRIMARY CARE

In this chapter I will identify some of the essential prerequisites for joint commissioning with GPs and Primary Care Teams and examine the challenges posed for Social Services Departments. Finally, a strategic framework for the development of joint commissioning between GPs and Social Services will be proposed.

There are a number of prerequisites for joint commissioning. Agencies have to trust each other, share common concerns, values and interests and without these prerequisites joint commissioning cannot really get started. There must be confidence in the other agency's management of resources before there is a willingness to share budgetary information, let alone any consideration of joint purchasing.

A number of face-to-face interviews with GPs in South West Hampshire during 1994 revealed that there was little trust or confidence in the Social Services Department and even less knowledge about their role in community care. GPs complained that access to Social Services Duty systems was difficult. One GP commenting on referrals to the Social Services Department said:

'I spend the morning trying to get through on the phone in between patients. I then give details and I often do not find out what is happening until I go to visit the patient.'

Many GPs said that when they made referrals to the Social

Services Department they did not hear the outcome. One GP had made a referral for one of his patients to go into residential care and said:

'The only reason I knew that she (patient) was not in residential care was because I saw her walking her dog.'

He had received no feedback about the assessment carried out by social services staff or the package of care delivered to support his patient in the community.

A number of GPs made comments about practice issues. One particular GP who served a number of residential care homes, the proprietors being his patients as well as their residents, alleged that:

'Social Services received backhanders to place people in some residential care homes.'

Another, perhaps less extreme view came from an inner city GP who said:

'A lot of money has gone to Social Services in recent years ... I would like to know what has happened to it.'

GPs had all received copies of the Community Care Plans but had rarely read them. One GP said of the Community Care Plan that:

'It was full of management speak and does not tell me about my patients needs.'

Finally, over half of the GPs interviewed confessed that they did not have enough information on community care. They wanted someone with whom they could have face-to-face contact on a regular basis and who could answer their questions as they arose. An examination of GP fundholders' 1993/94 purchasing plans made interesting reading. These plans are public documents and yet were rarely read by social services staff. The Health Authority asked all fundholders to comment on community care. One of the fundholders' plans read:

'Unfortunately in many instances, our contact with the Social Services Department takes place when patient management within the patient's home has reached a critical point, when arrangements for community care cannot be instigated immediately thus requiring hospital admission for the client.' (Bitterne Practice, Southampton)

Another had just three lines on community care:

'We make every effort to influence, support and work with Social Services and all our purchasing contracts require that the care programme approach should be used.' (Abbey Mead Practice, Romsey)

It is clear that we in the Social Services sector need to take steps to build up GPs trust, knowledge and confidence in our practice before joint commissioning can be effective.

One of the first challenges identified in trying to address these issues is the tension between the GPs generic responsibilities and the increasing moves of Social Services towards greater care group specialism.

GPs often asked for their 'own' care manager or social worker. Previous pilots where social workers had been placed into GPs surgeries had shown that smaller practices of four or less partners did not generate enough high priority work for a full time care manager or social worker. GPs need to access a wider range of services from the Social Services Department including child protection, mental health, visual and hearing impairment services, occupational therapy, domiciliary and residential care services. No one care manager could have the total range of skills needed to meet the needs of the primary care team.

By identifying one care manager to link to a particular surgery the Social Services Department could however, provide the familiar point of contact requested. The linked social worker could liaise with other social services staff to ensure that they gave feedback to particular GPs when a specialist response was needed. They could pick up non-urgent referrals to avoid all contacts having to be routed through the busy duty systems, and could provide up to date information on community care. After a year of having a linked worker the evaluation showed that trust and understanding of Social Services had improved.

One GP said:

'The link worker attends our primary care meetings and all referrals are discussed there. Consequently our referrals are more appropriate, our awareness of how to refer has increased, and the speed of action from Social Services has increased. Social Services are involved earlier and the whole team has benefited not just the GPs.'

The care manager on the other hand felt that the speed of action was the same, what had changed was the GPs awareness of what was happening.

The second challenge for Social Services Departments is the need to change our traditional pattern of seeking consultation by paper or large meetings. GPs are inundated with paperwork, most of which gets sorted by the practice manager and never reaches the GP. In addition they rarely attend meetings scheduled during surgery hours. The link worker's face-to-face contact provides a means of educating GPs about community care and obtaining their views about service developments. One of the GPs said, after a year of having access to a care manager:

'I have not sought to know all the ins and outs of community care although my awareness has inevitably increased; the important thing has been the resource of a person who has the information at their fingertips and to whom I can turn with confidence that they have the most up to date information possible.'

Thirdly, primary health care teams operate in very individual ways. It can be difficult for a Social Services Department to establish effective communications with GPs because of this diversity. In order for care managers to give feedback on the outcomes of referrals, communication systems need to be developed with each individual PHCT. The use of electronic mail, faxes and notebooks kept at the surgeries for GPs to make non-urgent referrals and for care managers to write outcomes, are some of the methods used to enhance communication. It is clear that as care managers work more closely with PHCTs and share information, there is reduced duplication of assessment and more efficient use of resources. A user interviewed as part of one of the primary care management pilot evaluations said that having a care manager attached to the practice had worked well for her:

'I started off talking about the future with my doctor, and I did not have to repeat all of this (to the care manager) when she came. I also think it stops people getting confused about what they are each supposed to be doing.'

Another user said of the care manager:

'She knew a lot more than the doctor and was at pains to explain what was possible. I think it is part of her job to have time to do this. What impressed me most was that she did not just stand there like a statue saying "Yes" to everything, which is what you get from so many people who do not know their stuff'.

There is no one model that will guarantee closer integration between primary health care teams and Social Services. The very individuality of each primary health care team means that a variety of models is needed. In some practices district nurses can be the focal point for all community care referrals. Their role can be enhanced by training them as care managers and allowing them access to funding for community care packages via the Social Services team manager. Five inner city practices with a high demand for community care services agreed to the use of Joint Finance money to pilot having two care managers to take all their referrals and to liaise with the local Social Services.

The final challenge to SSDs is how to develop joint commissioning with GPs and at the same time continue to ensure equity of service provision across the Social Services Department's area. GPs prime concern rests with the patients registered with their practice. The Social Services Department's public accountability via their elected members, means that they need to ensure that resources are used equitably across all primary care groupings. The more progressive GPs whose primary care services are often of the highest standard are also the ones who request access to their own care manager or involvement in a new pilot. What happens then about the single handed inner city practitioners who rarely refer to the Social Services Department? It is for this reason that SSD need to be proactive in developing links with GPs and not always wait for the approach to come from the Health Authorities or GPs themselves. Social services staff can target GPs whom they know to have patients with a high demand for community care services. In addition, it is essential that SSDs consistently apply their own eligibility criteria to ensure that there is equity in the distribution of resources.

By having team managers as budget holders SSDs are able to ensure that all care managers have equal access to the resources available, whether they be a district nurse, a care manager attached or linked to a primary care team, or an area office worker. By taking these steps Social Services Departments are more likely to secure equity.

Practice-level alliances

The framework proposed here for Social Services to develop joint commissioning with GPs relies on the essential link between practitioners, care managers and GPs. It is at this level that there are shared concerns and values: GPs with their individual patients and care managers with their clients or users. An understanding of each other's demands and priorities can lead to the exploration of shared interests, opportunities for reduction of service duplication, reinvestment into more effective practice and eventually joint purchasing and commissioning. This model suits those people who to date have not been the priority groups for joint commissioning; the huge numbers of elderly and disabled people who fill up the GPs' waiting rooms and care managers' case loads.

At the local level, team managers need to identify primary care teams in their area and to explore opportunities for developing working practices. Many team managers do not know the size or demographic make up of their local primary care teams: which GPs specialise in the care of the elderly or disabled, or which PHCTs cover local residential or nursing homes, for example. By starting with this basic fact finding, opportunities for closer working will become apparent. If Social Services Department local team managers take the lead then they can ensure that they target those practices with the greatest need. Having a range of options, such as linking workers to surgeries or training district nurses to be care managers, for example, makes negotiating with GPs easier. No one model will suit every practice. The importance of the team manager's role in supporting staff working with primary care, has to be stressed. Staff need to feel supported in applying Social Services' own eligibility criteria to ensure equity of service delivery. Some GPs have asked for the community care budgets to be devolved to primary care teams. How can equity be guaranteed across teams if this is the case? Is it that GPs have little confidence in Social Services' management of the budget because they receive so little feedback on how it is spent?

Aligning financial and service plans

In order to develop joint commissioning further once GPs and Social Services understand each other's demands and priorities and have developed a trusting working relationship, it will be important to examine community care budgets alongside fundholders' budgets. These can be aligned so that it becomes possible to examine more economical methods of purchasing whilst each agency still remains responsible for its own budget.

Finally, a good place to begin the process of examining the needs of a practice population is with the fundholders' purchasing plan. SSD local teams often have their own business plan covering the needs of their local population. Team managers should be encouraged to share their business plans with local GPs and to read fundholders' plans. It is possible to achieve a change in the GPs' perceptions of Social Services in a relatively short space of time. One of the practices wrote a year after having an attached care manager:

'We are particularly pleased with the development of the care manager project, and better links with Social Services have been established. The aims have been achieved with great success in improved communication and rapid and efficient management of problems. We can now work effectively to keep vulnerable people at home with support.' (Woolston Lodge Health Care Plan 1996/97)

A second practice noted that savings had been made and were considering reinvesting in care management themselves:

'The practice has been extremely pleased with the services provided by the attached social worker over the past 9 months. Unfortunately this pilot scheme is now coming to an end and the practice will have to review if monies from growth or savings should be used for employing social worker input. Patients in the community here had an efficient and early input at tapping social care provision and packages of care. The Southampton University Hospitals NHS Trust have had benefits by the reduction of admissions to acute beds.' (Bitterne Practice Health Care Plan 1996/97)

THE FUTURE CHALLENGE

Social Services Departments have begun to understand how essential it is for them to begin to examine joint commissioning with GPs in the light of the development of a Primary Care-Led NHS. There are many areas of common concern which once confidence and trust are established can lead to exciting opportunities for joint commissioning. The first step in this process is the link between care managers and GPs which needs to be established. Issues such as public accountability and equity for Social Services and the individualism of primary care need to be discussed openly and opportunities for joint commissioning placed firmly within this framework.

SOURCE DOCUMENTS

Abbey Mead (Romsey) Health Care Plan 1994/95
Bitterne Practice (Southampton) Health Care Plan 1994/95
Bitterne Practice (Southampton) Health Care Plan 1996/97
Department of Health 1994: Implementing Care For People: The Role Of The GP
    and Primary Health Care Team
Woolston Lodge (Southampton) Health Care Plan 1996/97

11. Managerial Effectiveness: The Wiltshire example

Yvonne Wilkin and Ralph Heywood

It is fitting that the last of the purely local case examples in this book should be Wiltshire. In terms of effectively combining health and social services in primary care, Wiltshire is arguably the national frontrunner in 1997. This chapter, therefore, can justifiably claim to offer others a methodology for the new style of management required in a much more diverse and devolved care system, based not on what is planned but on what has been achieved. Organisational and managerial effectiveness are especially closely related. There is, accordingly, much common ground between Southampton and Wiltshire, most obviously in their 'Linkworker' schemes which recognise that service interfaces themselves require dedicated management and organisational support. The Southampton Experience illustrates well the different stages of intra-organisational development required. The Wiltshire Experience goes further in pointing to the actual development of different types of organisation.

JOINT COMMISSIONING AT PRIMARY CARE LEVELS

In Wiltshire the purpose of the drive towards effective joint working in primary care is clear — to achieve the best possible service for users through the 'one stop shop' of primary care and by planning services together. We believe an integrated primary health and social care service can be more accessible, acceptable and locally responsive for users. The closer relationship between the General Practice and Social Services team is fundamental to a holistic approach to patients in the Primary Care-led NHS. As Pietroni[1] has pointed out this is 'Primary Care' and not 'Primary Health Care', and it represents a challenge for General Practice as well as for Social Services.

The management task in moving towards this is formidable and could not be accomplished without commitment and champions at the most senior level. Developments in Wiltshire during the 1990s have led to a range of models for joint working in the primary care setting.

Moving to mainstream — the Linkworker Scheme

The Social Care Linkworker Scheme started as a pilot in 1991 at six practices and has already been well documented.[2,3] By the end of 1996 there were 26 staff working with 53% of Wiltshire GPs. Their work combines care management and a development role. Linkworkers are joint funded and the scheme itself is the result of joint commissioning by the Social Services Department and the Health Authority. The expansion from the pilot phase was made possible by:

- Funding from the former FHSA and from the Special Transitional Grant for Community Care;
- The 'ripple effect' among GPs as the good word about the pilots passed on and practices put in bids for their own linkworker;
- Commitments from Social Services' Team Managers to make a contribution from their own staff complement.

Development staff input was required throughout the process. Social services' contact with practices, through linkworkers and named team staff, has now reached 'critical mass' so that the prospect of completing the process, including all willing practices, now looks feasible.

One of the challenges for Social Services' Team Managers was inequity caused by linkworkers being based at some General Practices and not others, and generating additional but 'lower priority' work. A number of practices also feel a lack of equity because they have been asking for a linkworker and do not yet have one. With the current limited resources in Social Services, and managers' concerns about how to fulfil such requirements as duty cover, further progress will be slow. However, it is helped by greater understanding on the part of GPs, so that the effort of reaching these new arrangements is not seen as one-way by the Social Services team.

The Linkworker Scheme, at the end of 5 years, is now mainstream and established within Adult Care Teams as well as many Primary Health Care Teams. Operational managers have had time to realise the commitment and vision of closer joint working, and this now has considerable momentum.

From linkworking to joint commissioning

The Linkworker Scheme has laid the foundation for a variety of joint commissioning projects at primary care level. Practice-based joint commissioning is defined in Wiltshire as 'a process which requires networking, local need, assessment, creative approaches to meeting those needs, and contracting and purchasing.'[4] These projects have been designed to enable local Social Services Teams and individual General Practices to focus on meeting the needs of specific groups.

Wiltshire Social Services Department has based workers in each of the participating practices and their role is to explore how joint care management can create a better coordinated approach for service users. The Wiltshire Children's Service Plan has been the catalyst for a number of joint initiatives, including using Joint Finance to employ linkworkers for children with disabilities in Trowbridge and Salisbury. The same approach has been taken with two practices in Swindon where a linkworker has explored the scope for developing preventive family support services from a general practice base.

Three projects have focused specifically on practice-based joint commissioning for mental health. Each practice team has been encouraged to develop its own objectives based on local assessments of need. The SSD has dedicated additional social work time to the projects which have sought to strengthen the links between primary care and specialist mental health services.

The longest running of the practice-based joint commissioning projects in the county began in 1993 in Trowbridge and Malmesbury and have concentrated on meeting the needs of older people and their carers. These projects formed part of the Kings Fund National Joint Community Care Commissioning Project[5] and are now providing models of how Social Services and general practice can, given the right conditions, form a strong alliance which transcends organisational boundaries for the benefit of their local population. The shared belief, as described in Chapter 5 and 6 of this book, is that the development of the joint commissioning of services for older people will be most effective if it is carried out at a very local level.

These two projects began in 1993 and have the ambitious aim of linking strategic joint commissioning between Social Services and the Health Authority with the operational purchasing being undertaken by Social Services Adult Care Teams working with colleagues in General Practice. It has inevitably taken some time for the key local players (Social Services Team Managers, General Practitioners and Practice Managers) to forge a shared understanding of what joint commissioning means for them and how to involve older people and carers in the work. From tentative beginnings, however, a strong partnership has grown and now the SSD and the two General Practices have combined their staff in integrated teams based in the Practices.

This means that the practice has truly become the focal point for the arrangement of community care services for its population and has the staff, resources and budgets which enable the practice based team to meet users' needs. Progress has seemed slow at times but it is hard to over-estimate the significance of what is being achieved through the establishment of an empowered local primary care team working alongside users and carers to commission community care based on a real knowledge and understanding of local needs.

THE MANAGERIAL CHALLENGES

What are the management issues raised by joint commissioning at primary care level?

User and carer expectations

Some users and carers see it as entirely natural that health and social services workers in contact with them share information and have a coordinated approach. They assume it happens and that it is to their benefit. Some users do not wish their social care services to be connected with their health care, and this may be due to concern that all their needs are being addressed under the 'medical model'. Increasingly, disabled people will be receiving direct payments and will manage their own care. Until there is a different type of primary care, not medically dominated, some people will wish to get their support elsewhere. This message has been heard in Wiltshire and the choice of channels for obtaining help will be maintained.

The development of GP Fundholding and commissioning has brought a new focus on the power and influence of GPs, yet there is concern about how democratic this is and how managing the money fits with the doctor-patient relationship.

Organisational and operational issues

The vision of integrated primary health and social care needs to be promoted at senior level, as it is in Wiltshire, but achieving change is notoriously difficult, not least amongst people working under pressure.

Whilst 'integration' is seen as highly positive for the service user, it represents possible disruption and even a threat for existing teams. The assumption is that the basic building block for the future is the General Practice, yet SSD teams work to the population in a given area, and are able to support and inform each other at their team base. Working to a GP list may cut across this, and the teams may not appreciate the primacy of the GP-patient relationship. After all, Social Services staff work with people when they have a need and then close the case.

In addition to reorganising workers to align with the practice population, with its associated risk of fragmentation, team managers have to adopt a different style for supporting outposted workers. To accept this, they need to be able to see and believe in the benefits. One way of doing this is to evaluate core work — care management — and try to identify benefits in terms of duplication avoided, time saved on gathering information and a smoother service for the user. And for the General Practice, there is a major difference between accommodating one or two additional SSD staff, sharing premises with a team of them in real partnership style, or getting involved in planning together. Both the Trowbridge and Malmesbury projects are, however, working through these issues with assistance from development and training staff.

Practice, or locality commissioning?

For specialist services, the individual practice may not be the appropriate commissioning unit. This is also the case for very small practices, but practices can collaborate for commissioning. Andrew Willis[6] is very positive about the benefits of GP commissioning, but emphasises that the appropriate population must be used for different services. Thus, commissioning may be at district level for more specialised services, at locality level for others and for some at practice level. The project on integrated commissioning for older people in Trowbridge involves all four practices in the town and, whilst recognising the individuality of practices, is also able to look towards service development for them all.

When aiming for closer working relationships with a scattering of single handed practices, Social Services Departments are stretched to use workers efficiently, though managers may try. In terms of prospects for joint commissioning, practices moving towards collaborating in groups will also create fertile territory for joint work with Social Services.

A GP-led organisation?

GPs have taken a lot on — or had it thrust upon them — but how prepared are they for the strategic tasks of analysing population need and specifying services, managing the ever more complex multi-disciplinary setting, and acting as part of a team? How publicly accountable are they for the large budgets they now control? These and other concerns have been expressed by Ray Jones,[7] and are in the minds of Social Services managers in Wiltshire. GPs and practices are extremely diverse and integrating with them is a test of confidence, especially as it consumes time and energy.

Working closely with practices is about current service, but is also about getting alongside the 'medical model' to help the shift towards something new. It is important to realise that GPs within the same Practice do not necessarily work as a team, and may not want to do more than their clinical work.

The pressures now operating on General Practice are causing a change in its dynamics. Professional practice management has become established, and other practice models, (e.g. salaried GPs) are now formally central policy.[8] In Wiltshire, developments are bringing the Social Services perspective into General Practice, and there is learning on both sides. This groundwork is part of the evolution of a new primary care which will serve health and social care needs holistically.

Managing diversity

The primary based joint commissioning projects represent a significant plank in the joint objective of the Health Authority and Social Services Department to 'work towards integration of social and primary health care services for commissioning and community care' (Wiltshire Community Care Plan). The time and support required to sustain the various projects is considerable. It has required dedicated staff time within both Health and Social Services agencies at senior level from people who have confidence and skills to move easily between the different organisational levels. The management task has been to enable GPs and Social Services Team Managers to lead the projects whilst guiding them around the potential pitfalls in bringing different bureaucratic systems together. The Social Services Department and the Health Authority operate within different structures for accountability and to different sets of rules.

However, this process builds mutual confidence and understanding on which significant and lasting service changes can be founded. An important lesson in Wiltshire has been the pivotal role that service users and their carers play in focusing local professionals on what really matters — their experience of services and how they think they can be improved. At the same time it has been important not to try to impose preconceived models of how joint commissioning at primary care level might be done. The framework for joint commissioning must be sufficiently loose to allow local players to shape direction and priorities but yet tight enough to avoid wasteful energy which will not gain support within the Health Authority and SSD.

The final lesson to managing diversity is that the GPs' involvement is vital. A key to success in Trowbridge and Malmesbury has been the enthusiasm of at least one GP in each practice whilst recognising that all the partners need to have some awareness of the projects and at least a tacit commitment to the benefits of strong collaborative working. There is no short cut.

Managing continuous change

The success of the developments in Wiltshire has been a combination of serendipity and sustained management commitment. From small beginnings the linkworking scheme has grown to a point where 65% of GPs in the county have a linkworker or a 'named' worker in their local Social Services team providing direct access for their patients to a range of community care services. A significant number of practices are now experimenting with joint commissioning in different forms including the provision of community care packages, integrated primary care teams, joint needs assessment, working together on practice plans, sharing information systems and so on.

The work was given an initial impetus through a joint development fund but has now reached the point when further development can only be sustained through the repatterning of existing resources. This poses a challenge and a threat to SSD managers and GPs who have seen the linkworker scheme as a growth in resources. It raises fundamental questions about how Social Services and General Practice are organised.

At this point in time some of these questions cannot be fully resolved and it is not clear how far Social Services Departments, Health Authorities and GPs can push boundaries within current organisational structures. What is clear, however, is that there is still plenty of scope for innovation and change, drawing on the experience which has been gained. The management challenge is to assimilate the lessons learnt into our different organisations in ways which change practice, structures and systems and to support moves in the direction of a primary care led service.

Joint purchasing

Wiltshire Social Services Department has devolved budget responsibility for purchasing community care services to local Team Managers. The average population covered by an Adult Care Team is 45 000 but ranges from 35 000 to nearly 70 000. Each team relates to between three and eight General Practices.

There is therefore considerable potential to move beyond agreement to buy care jointly for individuals and to commission service developments through combined purchasing arrangements. The response so far by fundholders to proposals to 'put money on the table' for joint commissioning is that they generally have little 'spare cash' or flexibility within the rules governing fundholding. However, there does appear to be greater scope within the Total Fundholding Project and a number of joint initiatives have been developed. These include joint purchasing of nursing home care to provide emergency and respite care as an alternative to admission to the local community hospital.

The management challenge is to find a way to enable fundholders, total fundholders, non-fundholders and SSD budget managers to use money jointly to resolve local problems and meet local needs. A first step is to remove some of the mystique surrounding budgets and who pays for what. This can be achieved within Social Services Departments by giving practices information about what is spent on their patients and what represents a 'fair share' of the Social Services budget for their population. This greater transparency about resources is a vital first step towards joint commissioning.

TOOLS OF THE TRADE

The picture that has been painted of diversity and local action is a challenge to Health and Local Authorities. The success of practice-based joint commissioning lies in the strong sense that individual linkworkers, social services team managers, GPs, practice managers and primary health team members, working alongside service users and carers, now have about being able to have a direct and personal influence on the way services are commissioned and provided. At a local level Health and Social Services staff do share a strong sense of common purpose. This can be successfully harnessed if the strategic authorities work together to encourage team work, to enable genuine participation in the decision making processes and to provide direct and practical assistance when difficulties arise.

The role of Social Services and Health Service Senior Managers is to provide the joint commissioners at primary care level with the tools of the trade.

Advice and guidance

These tools include clear and concise advice and guidance on what is permissible both to achieve the strategic aims of the authorities and to ensure probity and accountability. A handbook, *'Getting in Step — A Guide to Practice-based Joint Commissioning'* has been made available in Wiltshire to Social Services teams and all practices. This is a truly practical tool, incorporating key definitions which set out the purpose and benefits of joint commissioning and break the process into four steps which are then described and illustrated with examples from the projects in the county (Fig. 11.1). The four steps are:

- Creating local networks;
- Needs assessment;
- Service stimulation and specification;
- Contracting and purchasing.

Staff developments

This also involves using staff development training resources in ways which encourage shared understanding of care management and care planning in respect of the roles and responsibilities of different professionals. It demands a project management style which

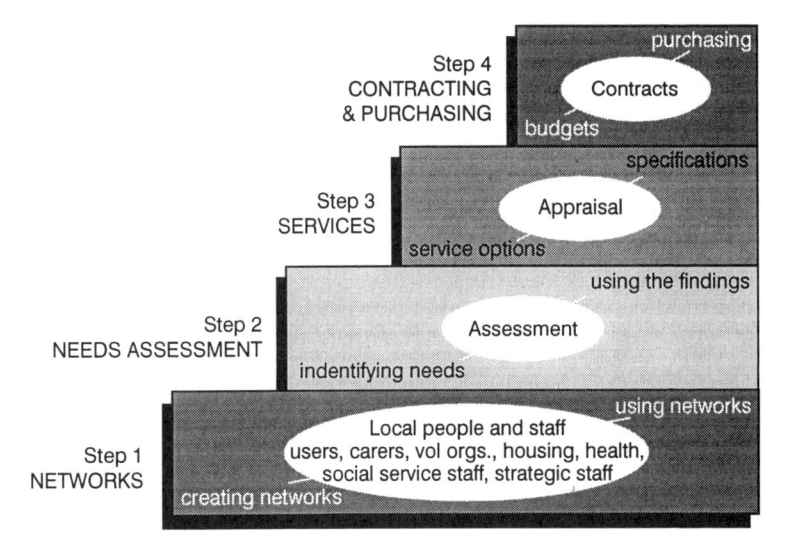

```
Step 4                      purchasing
CONTRACTING         Contracts
& PURCHASING
                     budgets
                                   specifications
    Step 3           Appraisal
   SERVICES
              service options
                            using the findings
  Step 2              Assessment
NEEDS ASSESSMENT
              indentifying needs
                                   using networks
              Local people and staff
  Step 1     users, carers, vol orgs., housing, health,
NETWORKS         social service staff, strategic staff
             creating networks
```

Fig. 11.1

enables joint commissioning to be broken down into its component steps so that the different players can understand their role within their local networks and how they can contribute to and influence the outcomes. Health and Social Services need to commit staff time to practice-based joint commissioning to ensure that it both retains a high profile alongside all the other management priorities and that there are champions within the organisation.

Creative pragmatism

Finally, 'creative pragmatism' is required, so that opportunities to bring Social Services and the Primary Health Care Teams closer together can be taken. In Wiltshire the creation of a new Health Authority and the disruption caused by Local Government Reorganisation could have been a barrier to progress. The uncertainty and instability caused by Wiltshire Health Authority transferring some of its population to Avon and the Local Authority being split into Swindon and the 'new' county might have led to a refocusing of management efforts and energies. In practice, however, it has provided opportunities for closer working. The Social Services Department has reorganised into smaller teams to strengthen links at a local level.

WHERE NEXT?

A key lesson from the joint commissioning work at practice level in Wiltshire is that the formation of these new relationships cannot be rushed. Time is needed to establish enduring local networks and to ensure that connections between the strategic aims of the commissioning authorities and the needs and priorities identified at a local level are shared and understood. Creating this shared agenda is an absolute prerequisite to future success. The lessons so far are that multi-disciplinary primary care teams working from a General Practice base are in a strong position to meet local needs and to use joint commissioning as a tool to bring about lasting improvements in services. There is much to be positive about in the achievements despite the financial pressures on both the Health and Local Authorities and the sometimes seemingly incompatible worlds of Social Services and General Practice.

The White Paper, *Choice and Opportunity*[8] has paved the way for even more radical changes in the way primary care services might be organised and delivered. It is possible to envisage a future where a range of organisations could set up and run local primary care centres. The experience from Wiltshire is that the drive towards integration of health and social care at this level will only be successful if time and support is given to enable the more subtle changes in joint working practices and inter-agency collaboration to be achieved.

REFERENCES

1. Pietroni P 1996 A Primary Care-led NHS — Trick or Treat? Purchasing in Practice 9
2. Jones R 1995 Moving towards integrated health and social care management. Primary Care Management 5(5)
3. Warner M, Macalister-Smith E 1996 Integrating health and social care. In: Meads G (ed) A Primary Care-Led NHS — Putting it into practice. Churchill Livingstone, Edinburgh
4. Challis L, Pearson J 1996 Getting in Step — A Guide to Practice-Based Joint Commissioning. Kings Fund, Wiltshire County Council, University of Bath
5. Poxton R 1996 A Better Old Age. Kings Fund, London
6. Willis A 1996 Commissioning — the best for all. In Littlejohns P, Victor C (Eds) Making sense of Primary Care-led Health Service. Radcliffe Medical Press, Oxford
7. Jones R 1996 Realizing the potential. Primary Care Management 6(7/8)
8. Department of Health 1996 Choice and Opportunity. Primary Care: the Future, HMSO, London

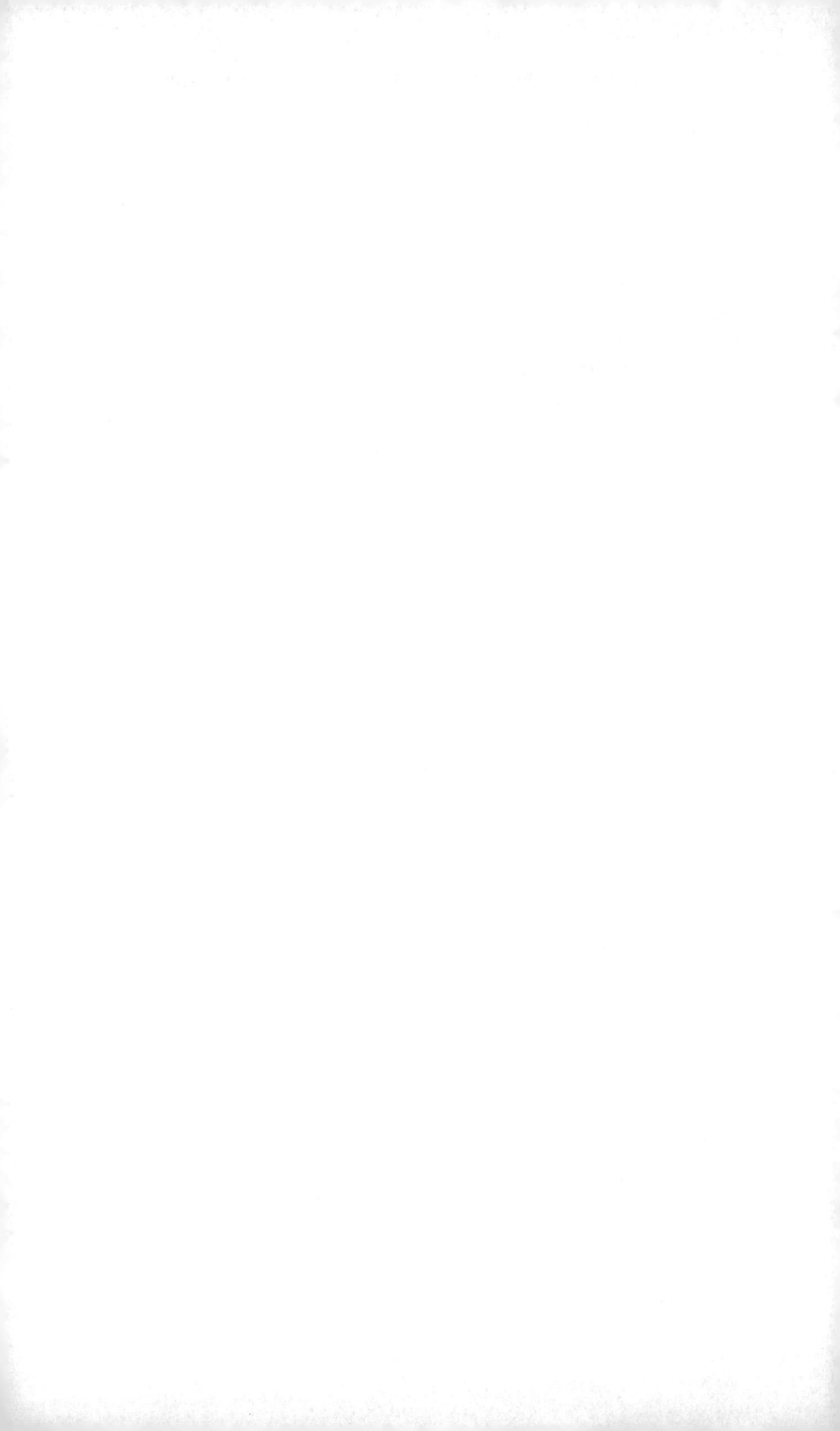

12. Personal Effectiveness: Charting icebergs — change below the surface

Andrew Webster

*This chapter rounds off the book both by completing the local case material and by further filling in the framework sketched out by Valerie Iles in Chapter 8. The role of its author, Andrew Webster, is a sign of the times: he is the Audit Commission's first Director of Joint Reviews (for Health and Social Services). Not so long ago somebody with Webster's planning background in both health and local authorities would, in all probability, have been consigned to 'liaison' tasks. He addresses the least fashionable but still most important dimension of the framework for effective combinations: personal effectiveness. The dissonance between values and behaviour can be particularly debilitating in the present decade, given the scale and speed of role changes for individuals and their motivation. Public services may no longer depend upon a consensus for their maintenance and development, and a calculated commitment is compatible with the more utilitarian approach. But it would be ironic indeed if the new focus on primary care, given its values in the UK, did not lead to a renewed consideration of what is right for **the person**, and what is needed to release the potential in individuals of the strengthened relationships that can derive from locating health and social services in primary care.*

'We need to talk about the work instinct, not the work ethic ... we need to imagine it as something going on instinctively, autonomously, like beer works, like bread works ...' James Hillman, 1983[1]

ON THE RIGHT TRACK

Ministers, councillors, directors and policy managers persistently echo the refrain 'let's not re-invent the wheel' only to find to their astonishment that other people's wheels do not run straight (or at all) on their roads. The main reason for this is that in borrowing policy and management models organisations frequently forget the implications for their people who are expected to make them work.

This chapter looks at five dimensions of the individual's propensity to change in order to build effective working partnerships. These are then mapped onto a matrix which enables one to map the potential for productive partnerships. The dynamics of change are illustrated by charting one 'virtuous' circle reinforcing positive collaboration and one 'vicious' circle which inhibits it. The chapter concludes by examining how best to promote virtuous circles of personal development and working practice.

Dimensions of change

Propensity to change in order to achieve better working practice, in collaboration with others, can be viewed in five possible dimensions:

- Motivation — the origins of an individual's commitment to a type of work, community of people (family, colleagues) or organisational purpose;
- Professionalism — the social and work centred identity of each individual both as they perceive themselves and as others perceive them;
- Partnership — the extent to which individuals, professions and organisations seek allies as a style of work and the degree of involvement of users within that style;
- Reflection and dialogue — the type of communication which takes place and the spaces which exist or are created for communication between individuals;
- Sense of history — the balance between righting past wrongs and creating future rights in individuals' minds and in professional and organisational cultures.

All of these factors are critically influenced by time. In setting policy goals and service targets it is the future that matters. Past performance is in the past and will not change. Nevertheless, individuals base their judgements about the present largely on immediate past experience. Hence, most judgements about the efficacy of a team, about the capacity of others to help or about the role of another profession or technique are based on what they have offered not on what they might offer.

WHERE ARE WE NOW?

In any navigation, the hardest part is working out where one is starting from. At sea this is now achievable at the press of a button to access a global network of satellites enabling anyone with a receiver to plot their position to within a few metres. Navigational techniques available in health and social care for charting organisational and personal change resemble ancient seafaring, reliant either on trusted sages who can read the stars (when there are no clouds), or on immensely complex mathematical tables incomprehensible to all but the trained expert.[2]

The equivalents of longitude and latitude in this model are assertiveness and approval. Put simply, the more assertive and approved an individual or group, the more capable of change and collaborative practice they are. It will be helpful therefore to assess, candidly and uncritically, the perceived assertiveness and approval ratings of key players in the system (Fig. 12.1).

These four archetypes are, of course, exaggerated and different individuals always combine a mix. Equally, people feel differently at different times. Nevertheless, because approval is conferred rather than self-generated, and because assertiveness is inherent as well as contextual, the scope for individuals and organisations to

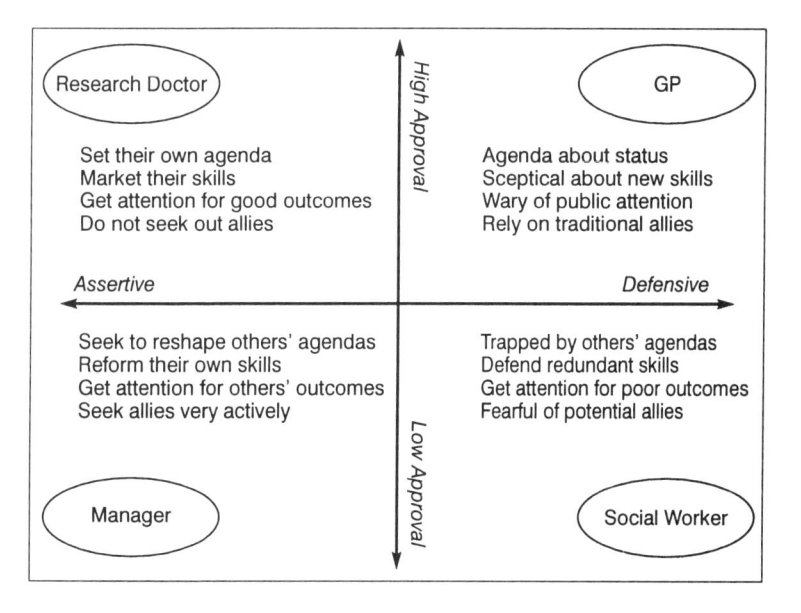

Assertive		Defensive
Research Doctor	*High Approval*	**GP**
Set their own agenda		Agenda about status
Market their skills		Sceptical about new skills
Get attention for good outcomes		Wary of public attention
Do not seek out allies		Rely on traditional allies
Seek to reshape others' agendas		Trapped by others' agendas
Reform their own skills		Defend redundant skills
Get attention for others' outcomes		Get attention for poor outcomes
Seek allies very actively		Fearful of potential allies
Manager	*Low Approval*	**Social Worker**

Fig. 12.1 Assertiveness/approval matrix

change their location on this matrix, in the short run, is small. Indeed it is probable that groups and professions change their location more as a result of changes in personnel than through changes in the outlook of existing members. Changes in social and political expectations can also have a powerful impact.

The contrasting experience of hospital administrators and social workers over the past 20 years illustrates this point. Since 1977 hospital administration has changed from balancing the power of unions and professions at the behest of uneasy alliances of local and national politicians into a group of managers who believe themselves, and are recognised by others, to exercise significant leadership in the NHS. Social Workers, on the other hand, have seen the emergent leadership in community development, personal empowerment and therapeutic communities turn into increasing uncertainty about purpose, skill and place in society. The primary driver of both changes was the reform of public services which greatly enhanced the role of resource management in the delivery of health and social care. Hospital administrators worked with measurable and therefore apparently more manageable resources (buildings, staff, laboratory tests, queues) while social workers work with intangible (though more valuable) resources of commitment, protection, mutual support and participation, the outcomes of which have not historically been deemed amenable to measurement.

It is apparent that joint practice between individuals with such different experience and characteristics provides the opportunity for everyone to draw on each others' strengths, and of course to fall out over each others' weaknesses. Two of the most common and inhibiting features of joint working are the tendency to ensure that no participant has much power, so that they cannot threaten others, and the tendency to exclude participants who would find this strategy insupportable. For example district nurses and home care workers might meet to reflect on how the time and energy put into planning complex support to a terminally ill person was wasted when the person's family prevailed on their GP to have them admitted to hospital. This is a mutually supportive exercise for district nurses and home carers, who share frustrations about carers and doctors but their reflection cannot alter the outcome. Earlier involvement of the family, and participation in care planning by the admitting hospital and the GP might have saved resources but would have brought deeper issues about the relationship with carers and medical staff into a space whose owners would prefer to exclude such powerful change drivers.

PERSONAL EFFECTIVENESS: CHARTING ICEBERGS 123

Since effective collaboration will require working with people and professional groups in all four quadrants of the assertiveness/approval matrix, the route to effectiveness is circular.

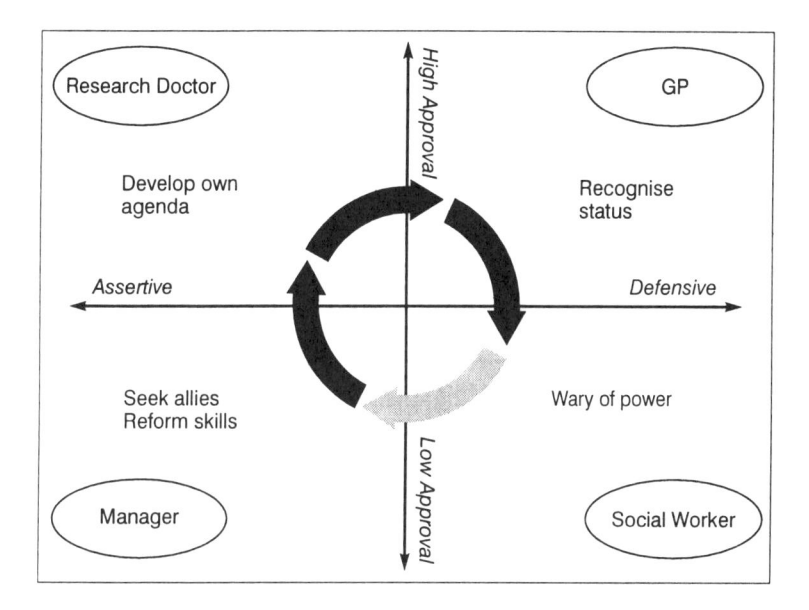

```
                    High Approval
                          ↑
   ( Research Doctor )    |    ( GP )

   Develop own            |    Recognise
   agenda                 |    status
                          |
   Assertive ─────────────┼───────────── Defensive
                          |
   Seek allies            |    Wary of power
   Reform skills          |
                          |
   ( Manager )            |    ( Social Worker )
                          ↓
                    Low Approval
```

Fig. 12.2 Promoting effectiveness

Charting the starting point using explicit judgements about status and attitude may be too challenging in a 'live' setting. In my experience inviting mixed groups of staff to use visual techniques like cartoons of one another or metaphors about day to day activities like gardening or housework can be powerful routes into establishing the same parameters. On one occasion a hospital doctor and social worker who worked closely together, though not harmoniously, both drew a cartoon of the other as a sly cat — make of that what you will!

Having set some markers it is important to identify potential change levers so that blocks or gaps can be addressed. Four candidates emerge from the dynamics of the matrix in Fig. 12.1:

- Interventions to help improve individuals' self-perception;
- Changes in status, rewards and public presentation which serve to improve individuals' sense of how others view them;
- Opportunties for people to explain their contribution positively to colleagues and peers;

- Set a common agenda about future achievables rather than previous obstacles.

Going round in the right direction

'It's impossible not to communicate. You cannot be for it or against it. You can only do it more or less well — by your own standards or by other people's — but you can't not do it.' Adam Phillips, 1996[3]

Effectiveness is best promoted when all four dimensions are addressed simultaneously. Focusing on users or clients becomes frustrating when no feedback is received and priorities are unclear. The more it is possible to work on all the drivers, the faster the circuit and the quicker is the progress to effective working.

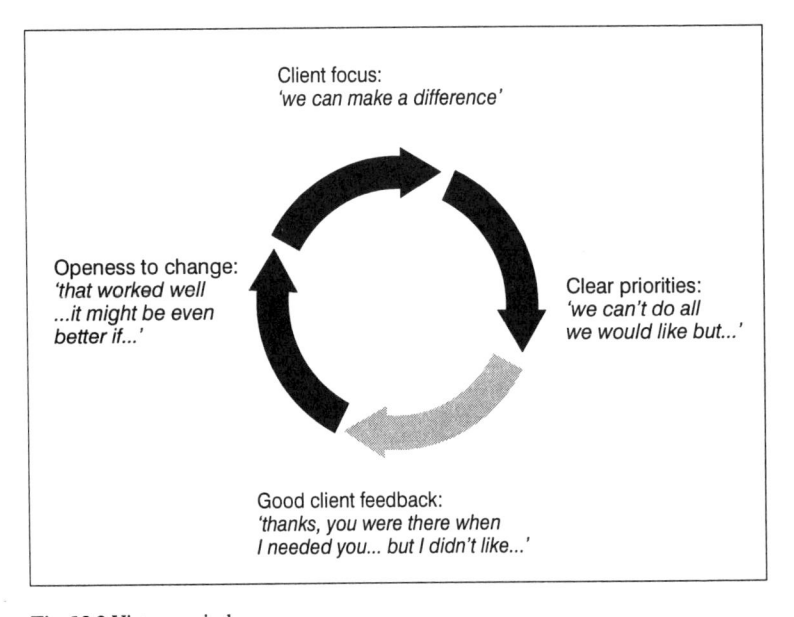

```
                Client focus:
                'we can make a difference'

Openess to change:                    Clear priorities:
'that worked well                     'we can't do all
 ...it might be even                   we would like but...'
 better if...'

                Good client feedback:
                'thanks, you were there when
                 I needed you... but I didn't like...'
```

Fig. 12.3 Virtuous circle

For example, primary care staff, social workers, independent providers, community mental health staff including psychiatrists and commissioners were able to work together in Clydebank (a community of 45 000 people on Clydeside just west of Glasgow), to establish a clear understanding that users' priorities were for a local, 24 hour, 7 day a week community oriented service which addressed the deficiencies of some existing residential care and provided more flexible access to support during the day. Priorities were set by targeting specific groups of severely ill and disabled people, by agreeing that the resettlement of 18 people in unsuitable accommodation would be a common goal and by developing a common understanding of the roles of the health centre and the mental health resource centre. Clients were encouraging in their willingness to contribute to setting up a local emergency response and in their comments about the improved service from the health centre and resource centre. Within a year primary care and social work professionals across a wide area saw Clydebank as an example of good practice.

Going in the wrong direction

'We can never be sure whether we are competing for something that doesn't exist, or winning a competition in which no one else is competing.'
Adam Phillips, 1996[4]

Equally, all four dimensions can feed a negative process which progressively reduces effectiveness. Where motivation and perceived status are driven by scapegoating outsiders, individuals, professions and organisations lose their focus on clients and have their poor performance confirmed and reinforced by poor feedback from users and peers.

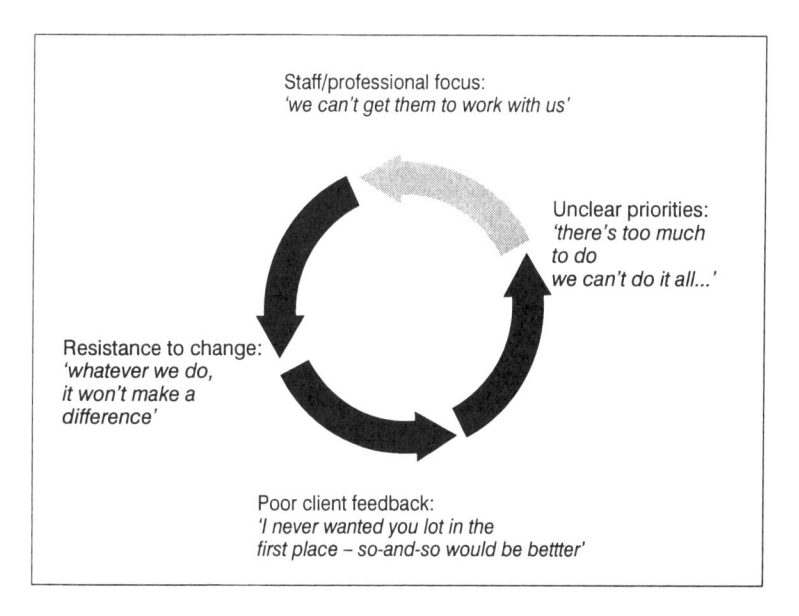

Fig. 12.4 Vicious circle

For example, in several instances poor outcomes for elderly people requiring residential care flow from ineffective relationships between primary care and social work. In one area team visited by the Audit Commission's Joint Review Team, understanding and user focus had declined to the point where GPs openly waited until weekends to make emergency placements in residential homes, or arranged emergency admissions into hospitals apparently to avoid the regular assessment process for social work support. This led to users being placed at short notice, with little or no choice, or undergoing unnecessary hospital admission, assessment and discharge often to access a service which they had not expressed a preference for. In some instances hospital stays were long enough, or their home circumstances fragile enough that an emergency decision by their GP foreclosed better options for their care.

General Practitioners were not happy with the situation which they recognised led to results which could not easily be defended and which also required considerable emergency work. The emergency social work service felt abused and responsible for failing to meet their Authority's commitments to users on assessment, participation and choice; naturally this led to resentment at the GPs who had occasioned this loss of professionalism. The local area social work team were mistrustful of primary care colleagues whom they perceived as waiting for an opportunity to bounce them into solutions they were incapable of undoing. No forum for addressing these issues existed except at Health Authority level, and relationships between GPs and the Health Authority, and between field social work staff and their strategic managers, were so distant that no capacity for facilitating better working could be envisaged by any participant in the process.

Managers and professionals in health and social care bemoan failure better than they celebrate success, so many readers will recognise the negative scenario and ask themselves the key question: *how do you change direction?*

Changing direction — dealing with the icebergs

Two features strike one immediately about both the virtuous and vicious circles. The same good and bad incentives are evident in both scenarios, and the kind of task, and work style required are the same. What distinguishes the virtuous from the vicious scenario, then? In these instances, and in many others, the essential differences appear to be that effective partnerships were built around agreed priorities for known users, that time to talk to users and with one another was consciously created, that local professionals and managers concerned themselves with the task in hand *and how it was performed*, that clearly achievable local targets were set and that these arrangements were endorsed and supported by strategic managers. In simple terms, individuals of different attitudes, motivations and professional backgrounds agreed what would be a good job in those specific circumstances, took time to check whether they were doing it and ensured that their bosses or stakeholders recognised and rewarded that good job.

A few simple initiatives can unlock the potential for a change in direction:

- Create some time and space for discussion of process separate from but linked to a common task;
- Give people individual incentives to work in a new partnerships including, for example, time off, development funding, administrative support;
- Go away — joint visits elsewhere won't show you too much new, but can make you look differently at 'home' and daily practice;
- Ask users what they think;
- Only enter into alliances if they have a purpose — be clear what it is;
- Set clear performance targets owned by local practitioners and top managers, stakeholders or politicians and measure them.

CONCLUSION

Many benefits for users and for individual workers can flow from changes in mind set, behaviour and systems which promote effectiveness and collaborative practice. Promoting change requires an honest appraisal of where individuals start from, recognition of different and evolving motivation, an acceptance of history as a basis for change and a clear process for reinforcing change through feedback and engagement with service users.

REFERENCES

1. Hillman J 1983 Interviews: Conversations Between James Hillman and Laura Pozzo on Therapy, Biography, Love, Soul, Dreams, Work, Imagination and the State of Culture. Harper and Row, New York
2. Sobel D 1996 Longitude. Fourth Estate, London
3. Phillips A 1996 Monogamy. Faber and Faber, London
4. Ibid

INDEX

Adult Care Teams
  linkworkers, 108
  populations covered, 114
Assertiveness/approval matrix, 121, 123
Audit Commission Joint Review Team, 126
Avon, transfer of population from Wiltshire, 116

Bath DHA, merger with Wiltshire FHSA, 50
Behaviours
  guardianship, 81
  trading, 81–2
  universally esteemed, 81
Bournemouth
  elderly people care in the community, 43–8
  evaluation issues, 43–4
  North Bournemouth, 44–6
  Southborne, 46–8

Care management, principles and process, 69
Case coordination, Cornwall system, 19–23
Change in initiatives, 126–7
Choice and generosity, 83–4
Choice and Opportunity, (White Paper), 117
Clydebank, 124–5
Communications, 75–86
  GPs and social workers, 76
  joint services in Southampton, 103
Community
  knowledge networks, heirarchy, 77–8
  problems, status, 78, 80–3
  ritualisation, 79–80
Community care, 4–5
  monitoring group, audit, 95
Community psychiatric nurses, Somerset, 89
Cornwall
  Care Management Model, 21
  case coordination, 19–23
  involvement of GPs, 19–23
  principal care system, 17–23

Discipline, levels, 84–5
Dorset Health Authority
  innovation in joint services, 42
  see also Poole; Trowbridge
Durham, Co
  joint services restructuring, 61–3
  Kings Fund Centre, Joint Commissioning Board, 64
  primary care strategy, 61–71
  primary care team, membership definitions, 36

Easington, Co Durham
  failures, 69–70
  future, 69–70
  Joint Commissioning Board, 64

Easington, Co Durham (*continued*)
Joint Commissioning Project model, 66–9
joint services model, 64–6
objectives, 67
'one stop shop', 64–5
primary care team development, 65–6
Effectiveness matrix, 123
Elderly people, care in the community
Bournemouth, 43–8
Trowbridge, 49–60

Fear, 85

Generosity, levels, 83–4
Getting in step – practice-based joint commissioning, Wiltshire, 115–16
GP fundholding
disadvantages, 9–11
purchasing plans, 101
Wiltshire, purchasing, 52–3
GPs
involvement, Cornwall system, 19–23
sharing of care managers, 103

Hampshire
closure of long stay hospitals, 99–100
Southampton organisation effectiveness, 99–106
see also Bournemouth; Southampton
Hayes
health plan, 29, 25–39
information, 27–9
Listening Exercise, 30–5
recurring themes, 34–5
location map, 28
political sensitivities, 33–4
primary care, 35–8
acute hospital services, 37–8
clinics, 36–7
GPs, 35–6
local ambulance sevices, 38
primary care team
building exercise, 33
consultation exercise, 32
resource usage, 29–30
Townfield Road profile, 31
see also London Borough of Hillingdon
Health, WHO definition, 75
Health potentials, knowledge networks heirarchy, 76–8
Health and social services
efficient combinations, 83–5
see also Joint services
Hillingdon *see* London Borough of Hillingdon
Hospital administrators role, 122

Initiatives, change, 126–7
Integrated health/social services care *see* Joint services

Jarman Index, 41–2
Joint commissioning, managerial challenges, 110–14
Joint Commissioning Board, Easington, Co Durham, 64
Joint Commissioning Project, Easington, Co Durham, 66–9
Joint services
commmunity care, principles, 94
convergence, advantages, 6–7, 7
efficient combinations, 83–5
hospital administrators role, 122
linkworking, 50–1
PC-led NHS, 9
purchaser/provider split, 62

Kings Fund, Trowbridge, Lovemead Group Practice, 53–5
Kings Fund Centre, Durham, Joint Commissioning Board, 64

Kings Fund National Joint Community Care, Commissioning Project, Trowbridge, 109
Knowledge network hierarchy, community, 77–8

Learning Disabilities Strategy audit, Somerset, 94–5
Somerset, 93–4
Linkworkers
  Adult Care Teams, 108
  inequity, 108
  joint commissioning, 109–10
  joint services, 50–1
  Southampton, 102
  Wiltshire
    numbers, 113
    schemes, 108–10
Linkworking, Wiltshire, practice-based assessment of commission, 50–1
London Borough of Hillingdon, 28–39
  anti-poverty programme, 26
  Mount View Hospital, multiagency consultation exercise, 32
  NHS trusts, 26
  Primary Care Listening Exercise, 32–5
  purchasing pilot scheme, 26
  see also Hayes
Lovemead Group Practice *see* Trowbridge

Management frameworks, 75
Managerial effectiveness, Wiltshire, 107–17
Mental Illness Specific Grant, 92
Monitoring group, community care, audit, 95
Motivation, 120
Multiagency partnerships, 25–6

NHS Act (1977), Section 28A (Joint Finance), 58

Nuffield Institute for Health, Easington, Co Durham, 66–7
Nurse assessors, Somerset, 89
Nursing care budget, Somerset, 91–2

Organisational boundaries, status, 80–1

Partnership, 120
Personal effectiveness, 119–27
  dynamics of change, 112–27
Poole, joint services project, 43
Primary care
  GPs part, 112
  management diversity and continuous change, 113–14
  organisation and operation issues, 111
  practice and locality communities, 111–12
  user and carer expectations, Wiltshire, 110–11
Primary Care Act (1997), 6
Primary care tasks, transfer of information, 79–80
Primary care-led NHS
  joint services, 9
  potential advantages, 9–10
  problems with GP fundholding, 10–11
  proposed model, 12–13
Professionalism, 120
Purchaser/provider separation
  joint services, 62
  Somerset, 92–5

Reflection and dialogue, 120
Resource usage, Hayes, 29–30
Responsibility, 84

Sense of history, 120
Somerset, 87–98
  community care legislation, 88–90
  contacts between joint services, 88

Somerset (*continued*)
  devolved budgets, 90–2
  fundholding, 88–9
  GPs, morbidity project, 98
  home care, 92
  hospital interfaces, 96–7
  Learning Disabilities Strategy, 93–4
  local responsibilities, 90–2
  MA/GP links, 98
  nurse assessors, 89
  nursing care budget, 91–2
  old peoples homes, 92
  primary care contingency plans, 77–8
  primary care deficit, 95–6
  purchaser/provider separation, 92–5
  research, 87–98
  UFM communities, 98
Somerset research, 87–98
  audit, Learning Disabilities Strategy, 94–5
Southampton, 99–106
  aligning financial and joint services plans, 103–4
  aligning financial and service plans, 8, 105–6
  care management, 105–6
  joint community
    four prerequisites, 100–6
    involvement of GPs and PHCTs, 99–100
    practice level alliances, 104–5
    primary care led purchasing, 99–100
  University Hospital NHS trust, benefits from joint services, 106
Status, community problems, 78, 80–3

Trading behaviours, 81–2
Trowbridge
  elderly people, care in the community, 49–60
  fundholding, 50
  Kings Fund National Joint Community Care, Commissioning Project, 109
Trowbridge, Lovemead Group Practice
  Affordable Domestic Assistance (ADA), 55
  contracting and commissioning, 57–8
  fundholding, 52–3
  future development, 59–60
  Handihelp West Wiltshire, 54–5
  Health and Social Care Team, 55–7
  Kings Fund, 53–5
  linkworker, 51–2
  practice general manager, 58
  Primary Care Liaison Management, 53
  and Social Services Adult Care Team
    joint services, 53–5
    New Services, 54–5
    specific initiatives, 59

Vicious circle, 124
Virtuous circle, 124

Wiltshire
  Children Services Plan, 109
  creative pragmatism, 116
  elderly people care in the community, joint services approach, 49
  joint purchasing, 114
  linkworker numbers, 113
  linkworker schemes, 108–10
  Lovemead practice *see* Trowbridge
  managerial effectiveness, 107–17
  'one stop shop', 107–8
  primary care-led purchasing, 52–3

Wiltshire (*continued*)
  social services/GP, joint services
    link worker, 50
    staff developments, 115–16
    transfer of population to Avon, 116
    user and carer expectations,
      primary care, 110–11
  see also Trowbridge
Wiltshire FHSA
  merger with Bath DHA, 50
  practice-based assessment of commission, 50–1